> TAKE CARE OF YOUR BODY.
> ITS THE ONLY PLACE YOU
> HAVE TO LIVE IN.

BLOOD SUGAR
AND
BLOOD PRESSURE
LOG BOOK

Name:_____

Address:_____
_____

Phone:_____

Email:_____

Blood Type:_____

Month: _____ **Week Commencing:** _____

Date __/__/__	BREAKFAST		LUNCH		DINNER		BEDTIME	
Monday	BEFORE	AFTER	BEFORE	AFTER	BEFORE	AFTER	BEFORE	AFTER
BLOOD SUGAR								
BLOOD PRESSURE								
Date __/__/__	BREAKFAST		LUNCH		DINNER		BEDTIME	
Tuesday	BEFORE	AFTER	BEFORE	AFTER	BEFORE	AFTER	BEFORE	AFTER
BLOOD SUGAR								
BLOOD PRESSURE								
Date __/__/__	BREAKFAST		LUNCH		DINNER		BEDTIME	
Wednesday	BEFORE	AFTER	BEFORE	AFTER	BEFORE	AFTER	BEFORE	AFTER
BLOOD SUGAR								
BLOOD PRESSURE								
Date __/__/__	BREAKFAST		LUNCH		DINNER		BEDTIME	
Thursday	BEFORE	AFTER	BEFORE	AFTER	BEFORE	AFTER	BEFORE	AFTER
BLOOD SUGAR								
BLOOD PRESSURE								
Date __/__/__	BREAKFAST		LUNCH		DINNER		BEDTIME	
Friday	BEFORE	AFTER	BEFORE	AFTER	BEFORE	AFTER	BEFORE	AFTER
BLOOD SUGAR								
BLOOD PRESSURE								
Date __/__/__	BREAKFAST		LUNCH		DINNER		BEDTIME	
Saturday	BEFORE	AFTER	BEFORE	AFTER	BEFORE	AFTER	BEFORE	AFTER
BLOOD SUGAR								
BLOOD PRESSURE								
Date __/__/__	BREAKFAST		LUNCH		DINNER		BEDTIME	
Sunday	BEFORE	AFTER	BEFORE	AFTER	BEFORE	AFTER	BEFORE	AFTER
BLOOD SUGAR								
BLOOD PRESSURE								

NOTES: _____
_____
_____
_____

Month: _____ Week Commencing: _____

Date __/__/__	BREAKFAST		LUNCH		DINNER		BEDTIME	
Monday	BEFORE	AFTER	BEFORE	AFTER	BEFORE	AFTER	BEFORE	AFTER
BLOOD SUGAR								
BLOOD PRESSURE								

Date __/__/__	BREAKFAST		LUNCH		DINNER		BEDTIME	
Tuesday	BEFORE	AFTER	BEFORE	AFTER	BEFORE	AFTER	BEFORE	AFTER
BLOOD SUGAR								
BLOOD PRESSURE								

Date __/__/__	BREAKFAST		LUNCH		DINNER		BEDTIME	
Wednesday	BEFORE	AFTER	BEFORE	AFTER	BEFORE	AFTER	BEFORE	AFTER
BLOOD SUGAR								
BLOOD PRESSURE								

Date __/__/__	BREAKFAST		LUNCH		DINNER		BEDTIME	
Thursday	BEFORE	AFTER	BEFORE	AFTER	BEFORE	AFTER	BEFORE	AFTER
BLOOD SUGAR								
BLOOD PRESSURE								

Date __/__/__	BREAKFAST		LUNCH		DINNER		BEDTIME	
Friday	BEFORE	AFTER	BEFORE	AFTER	BEFORE	AFTER	BEFORE	AFTER
BLOOD SUGAR								
BLOOD PRESSURE								

Date __/__/__	BREAKFAST		LUNCH		DINNER		BEDTIME	
Saturday	BEFORE	AFTER	BEFORE	AFTER	BEFORE	AFTER	BEFORE	AFTER
BLOOD SUGAR								
BLOOD PRESSURE								

Date __/__/__	BREAKFAST		LUNCH		DINNER		BEDTIME	
Sunday	BEFORE	AFTER	BEFORE	AFTER	BEFORE	AFTER	BEFORE	AFTER
BLOOD SUGAR								
BLOOD PRESSURE								

NOTES: _____

_____

_____

_____

Month: _____ **Week Commencing:** _____

Date __/__/__	BREAKFAST		LUNCH		DINNER		BEDTIME	
Monday	BEFORE	AFTER	BEFORE	AFTER	BEFORE	AFTER	BEFORE	AFTER
BLOOD SUGAR								
BLOOD PRESSURE								
Date __/__/__	BREAKFAST		LUNCH		DINNER		BEDTIME	
Tuesday	BEFORE	AFTER	BEFORE	AFTER	BEFORE	AFTER	BEFORE	AFTER
BLOOD SUGAR								
BLOOD PRESSURE								
Date __/__/__	BREAKFAST		LUNCH		DINNER		BEDTIME	
Wednesday	BEFORE	AFTER	BEFORE	AFTER	BEFORE	AFTER	BEFORE	AFTER
BLOOD SUGAR								
BLOOD PRESSURE								
Date __/__/__	BREAKFAST		LUNCH		DINNER		BEDTIME	
Thursday	BEFORE	AFTER	BEFORE	AFTER	BEFORE	AFTER	BEFORE	AFTER
BLOOD SUGAR								
BLOOD PRESSURE								
Date __/__/__	BREAKFAST		LUNCH		DINNER		BEDTIME	
Friday	BEFORE	AFTER	BEFORE	AFTER	BEFORE	AFTER	BEFORE	AFTER
BLOOD SUGAR								
BLOOD PRESSURE								
Date __/__/__	BREAKFAST		LUNCH		DINNER		BEDTIME	
Saturday	BEFORE	AFTER	BEFORE	AFTER	BEFORE	AFTER	BEFORE	AFTER
BLOOD SUGAR								
BLOOD PRESSURE								
Date __/__/__	BREAKFAST		LUNCH		DINNER		BEDTIME	
Sunday	BEFORE	AFTER	BEFORE	AFTER	BEFORE	AFTER	BEFORE	AFTER
BLOOD SUGAR								
BLOOD PRESSURE								

NOTES: _____
_____
_____
_____

Month: _____ **Week Commencing:** _____

Date __/__/__	BREAKFAST		LUNCH		DINNER		BEDTIME	
Monday	BEFORE	AFTER	BEFORE	AFTER	BEFORE	AFTER	BEFORE	AFTER
BLOOD SUGAR								
BLOOD PRESSURE								

Date __/__/__	BREAKFAST		LUNCH		DINNER		BEDTIME	
Tuesday	BEFORE	AFTER	BEFORE	AFTER	BEFORE	AFTER	BEFORE	AFTER
BLOOD SUGAR								
BLOOD PRESSURE								

Date __/__/__	BREAKFAST		LUNCH		DINNER		BEDTIME	
Wednesday	BEFORE	AFTER	BEFORE	AFTER	BEFORE	AFTER	BEFORE	AFTER
BLOOD SUGAR								
BLOOD PRESSURE								

Date __/__/__	BREAKFAST		LUNCH		DINNER		BEDTIME	
Thursday	BEFORE	AFTER	BEFORE	AFTER	BEFORE	AFTER	BEFORE	AFTER
BLOOD SUGAR								
BLOOD PRESSURE								

Date __/__/__	BREAKFAST		LUNCH		DINNER		BEDTIME	
Friday	BEFORE	AFTER	BEFORE	AFTER	BEFORE	AFTER	BEFORE	AFTER
BLOOD SUGAR								
BLOOD PRESSURE								

Date __/__/__	BREAKFAST		LUNCH		DINNER		BEDTIME	
Saturday	BEFORE	AFTER	BEFORE	AFTER	BEFORE	AFTER	BEFORE	AFTER
BLOOD SUGAR								
BLOOD PRESSURE								

Date __/__/__	BREAKFAST		LUNCH		DINNER		BEDTIME	
Sunday	BEFORE	AFTER	BEFORE	AFTER	BEFORE	AFTER	BEFORE	AFTER
BLOOD SUGAR								
BLOOD PRESSURE								

NOTES: _____
_____
_____
_____

Month: _____ Week Commencing: _____

Date __/__/__	BREAKFAST		LUNCH		DINNER		BEDTIME	
Monday	BEFORE	AFTER	BEFORE	AFTER	BEFORE	AFTER	BEFORE	AFTER
BLOOD SUGAR								
BLOOD PRESSURE								
Date __/__/__	BREAKFAST		LUNCH		DINNER		BEDTIME	
Tuesday	BEFORE	AFTER	BEFORE	AFTER	BEFORE	AFTER	BEFORE	AFTER
BLOOD SUGAR								
BLOOD PRESSURE								
Date __/__/__	BREAKFAST		LUNCH		DINNER		BEDTIME	
Wednesday	BEFORE	AFTER	BEFORE	AFTER	BEFORE	AFTER	BEFORE	AFTER
BLOOD SUGAR								
BLOOD PRESSURE								
Date __/__/__	BREAKFAST		LUNCH		DINNER		BEDTIME	
Thursday	BEFORE	AFTER	BEFORE	AFTER	BEFORE	AFTER	BEFORE	AFTER
BLOOD SUGAR								
BLOOD PRESSURE								
Date __/__/__	BREAKFAST		LUNCH		DINNER		BEDTIME	
Friday	BEFORE	AFTER	BEFORE	AFTER	BEFORE	AFTER	BEFORE	AFTER
BLOOD SUGAR								
BLOOD PRESSURE								
Date __/__/__	BREAKFAST		LUNCH		DINNER		BEDTIME	
Saturday	BEFORE	AFTER	BEFORE	AFTER	BEFORE	AFTER	BEFORE	AFTER
BLOOD SUGAR								
BLOOD PRESSURE								
Date __/__/__	BREAKFAST		LUNCH		DINNER		BEDTIME	
Sunday	BEFORE	AFTER	BEFORE	AFTER	BEFORE	AFTER	BEFORE	AFTER
BLOOD SUGAR								
BLOOD PRESSURE								

NOTES: _____
_____
_____
_____

Month: _____ **Week Commencing:** _____

Date __/__/__	BREAKFAST		LUNCH		DINNER		BEDTIME	
Monday	BEFORE	AFTER	BEFORE	AFTER	BEFORE	AFTER	BEFORE	AFTER
BLOOD SUGAR								
BLOOD PRESSURE								
Date __/__/__	BREAKFAST		LUNCH		DINNER		BEDTIME	
Tuesday	BEFORE	AFTER	BEFORE	AFTER	BEFORE	AFTER	BEFORE	AFTER
BLOOD SUGAR								
BLOOD PRESSURE								
Date __/__/__	BREAKFAST		LUNCH		DINNER		BEDTIME	
Wednesday	BEFORE	AFTER	BEFORE	AFTER	BEFORE	AFTER	BEFORE	AFTER
BLOOD SUGAR								
BLOOD PRESSURE								
Date __/__/__	BREAKFAST		LUNCH		DINNER		BEDTIME	
Thursday	BEFORE	AFTER	BEFORE	AFTER	BEFORE	AFTER	BEFORE	AFTER
BLOOD SUGAR								
BLOOD PRESSURE								
Date __/__/__	BREAKFAST		LUNCH		DINNER		BEDTIME	
Friday	BEFORE	AFTER	BEFORE	AFTER	BEFORE	AFTER	BEFORE	AFTER
BLOOD SUGAR								
BLOOD PRESSURE								
Date __/__/__	BREAKFAST		LUNCH		DINNER		BEDTIME	
Saturday	BEFORE	AFTER	BEFORE	AFTER	BEFORE	AFTER	BEFORE	AFTER
BLOOD SUGAR								
BLOOD PRESSURE								
Date __/__/__	BREAKFAST		LUNCH		DINNER		BEDTIME	
Sunday	BEFORE	AFTER	BEFORE	AFTER	BEFORE	AFTER	BEFORE	AFTER
BLOOD SUGAR								
BLOOD PRESSURE								

NOTES: _____

_____

_____

_____

Month: _____ **Week Commencing:** _____

Date __/__/__	BREAKFAST		LUNCH		DINNER		BEDTIME	
Monday	BEFORE	AFTER	BEFORE	AFTER	BEFORE	AFTER	BEFORE	AFTER
BLOOD SUGAR								
BLOOD PRESSURE								
Date __/__/__	BREAKFAST		LUNCH		DINNER		BEDTIME	
Tuesday	BEFORE	AFTER	BEFORE	AFTER	BEFORE	AFTER	BEFORE	AFTER
BLOOD SUGAR								
BLOOD PRESSURE								
Date __/__/__	BREAKFAST		LUNCH		DINNER		BEDTIME	
Wednesday	BEFORE	AFTER	BEFORE	AFTER	BEFORE	AFTER	BEFORE	AFTER
BLOOD SUGAR								
BLOOD PRESSURE								
Date __/__/__	BREAKFAST		LUNCH		DINNER		BEDTIME	
Thursday	BEFORE	AFTER	BEFORE	AFTER	BEFORE	AFTER	BEFORE	AFTER
BLOOD SUGAR								
BLOOD PRESSURE								
Date __/__/__	BREAKFAST		LUNCH		DINNER		BEDTIME	
Friday	BEFORE	AFTER	BEFORE	AFTER	BEFORE	AFTER	BEFORE	AFTER
BLOOD SUGAR								
BLOOD PRESSURE								
Date __/__/__	BREAKFAST		LUNCH		DINNER		BEDTIME	
Saturday	BEFORE	AFTER	BEFORE	AFTER	BEFORE	AFTER	BEFORE	AFTER
BLOOD SUGAR								
BLOOD PRESSURE								
Date __/__/__	BREAKFAST		LUNCH		DINNER		BEDTIME	
Sunday	BEFORE	AFTER	BEFORE	AFTER	BEFORE	AFTER	BEFORE	AFTER
BLOOD SUGAR								
BLOOD PRESSURE								

NOTES: _____
_____
_____
_____

Month: _____ Week Commencing: _____

Date __/__/__	BREAKFAST		LUNCH		DINNER		BEDTIME	
Monday	BEFORE	AFTER	BEFORE	AFTER	BEFORE	AFTER	BEFORE	AFTER
BLOOD SUGAR								
BLOOD PRESSURE								
Date __/__/__	BREAKFAST		LUNCH		DINNER		BEDTIME	
Tuesday	BEFORE	AFTER	BEFORE	AFTER	BEFORE	AFTER	BEFORE	AFTER
BLOOD SUGAR								
BLOOD PRESSURE								
Date __/__/__	BREAKFAST		LUNCH		DINNER		BEDTIME	
Wednesday	BEFORE	AFTER	BEFORE	AFTER	BEFORE	AFTER	BEFORE	AFTER
BLOOD SUGAR								
BLOOD PRESSURE								
Date __/__/__	BREAKFAST		LUNCH		DINNER		BEDTIME	
Thursday	BEFORE	AFTER	BEFORE	AFTER	BEFORE	AFTER	BEFORE	AFTER
BLOOD SUGAR								
BLOOD PRESSURE								
Date __/__/__	BREAKFAST		LUNCH		DINNER		BEDTIME	
Friday	BEFORE	AFTER	BEFORE	AFTER	BEFORE	AFTER	BEFORE	AFTER
BLOOD SUGAR								
BLOOD PRESSURE								
Date __/__/__	BREAKFAST		LUNCH		DINNER		BEDTIME	
Saturday	BEFORE	AFTER	BEFORE	AFTER	BEFORE	AFTER	BEFORE	AFTER
BLOOD SUGAR								
BLOOD PRESSURE								
Date __/__/__	BREAKFAST		LUNCH		DINNER		BEDTIME	
Sunday	BEFORE	AFTER	BEFORE	AFTER	BEFORE	AFTER	BEFORE	AFTER
BLOOD SUGAR								
BLOOD PRESSURE								

NOTES: _____
_____
_____
_____

Month: _____ **Week Commencing:** _____

Date __/__/__	BREAKFAST		LUNCH		DINNER		BEDTIME	
Monday	BEFORE	AFTER	BEFORE	AFTER	BEFORE	AFTER	BEFORE	AFTER
BLOOD SUGAR								
BLOOD PRESSURE								
Date __/__/__	BREAKFAST		LUNCH		DINNER		BEDTIME	
Tuesday	BEFORE	AFTER	BEFORE	AFTER	BEFORE	AFTER	BEFORE	AFTER
BLOOD SUGAR								
BLOOD PRESSURE								
Date __/__/__	BREAKFAST		LUNCH		DINNER		BEDTIME	
Wednesday	BEFORE	AFTER	BEFORE	AFTER	BEFORE	AFTER	BEFORE	AFTER
BLOOD SUGAR								
BLOOD PRESSURE								
Date __/__/__	BREAKFAST		LUNCH		DINNER		BEDTIME	
Thursday	BEFORE	AFTER	BEFORE	AFTER	BEFORE	AFTER	BEFORE	AFTER
BLOOD SUGAR								
BLOOD PRESSURE								
Date __/__/__	BREAKFAST		LUNCH		DINNER		BEDTIME	
Friday	BEFORE	AFTER	BEFORE	AFTER	BEFORE	AFTER	BEFORE	AFTER
BLOOD SUGAR								
BLOOD PRESSURE								
Date __/__/__	BREAKFAST		LUNCH		DINNER		BEDTIME	
Saturday	BEFORE	AFTER	BEFORE	AFTER	BEFORE	AFTER	BEFORE	AFTER
BLOOD SUGAR								
BLOOD PRESSURE								
Date __/__/__	BREAKFAST		LUNCH		DINNER		BEDTIME	
Sunday	BEFORE	AFTER	BEFORE	AFTER	BEFORE	AFTER	BEFORE	AFTER
BLOOD SUGAR								
BLOOD PRESSURE								

NOTES: _____

_____

_____

Month: _____ **Week Commencing:** _____

Date __/__/__	BREAKFAST		LUNCH		DINNER		BEDTIME	
Monday	BEFORE	AFTER	BEFORE	AFTER	BEFORE	AFTER	BEFORE	AFTER
BLOOD SUGAR								
BLOOD PRESSURE								
Date __/__/__	BREAKFAST		LUNCH		DINNER		BEDTIME	
Tuesday	BEFORE	AFTER	BEFORE	AFTER	BEFORE	AFTER	BEFORE	AFTER
BLOOD SUGAR								
BLOOD PRESSURE								
Date __/__/__	BREAKFAST		LUNCH		DINNER		BEDTIME	
Wednesday	BEFORE	AFTER	BEFORE	AFTER	BEFORE	AFTER	BEFORE	AFTER
BLOOD SUGAR								
BLOOD PRESSURE								
Date __/__/__	BREAKFAST		LUNCH		DINNER		BEDTIME	
Thursday	BEFORE	AFTER	BEFORE	AFTER	BEFORE	AFTER	BEFORE	AFTER
BLOOD SUGAR								
BLOOD PRESSURE								
Date __/__/__	BREAKFAST		LUNCH		DINNER		BEDTIME	
Friday	BEFORE	AFTER	BEFORE	AFTER	BEFORE	AFTER	BEFORE	AFTER
BLOOD SUGAR								
BLOOD PRESSURE								
Date __/__/__	BREAKFAST		LUNCH		DINNER		BEDTIME	
Saturday	BEFORE	AFTER	BEFORE	AFTER	BEFORE	AFTER	BEFORE	AFTER
BLOOD SUGAR								
BLOOD PRESSURE								
Date __/__/__	BREAKFAST		LUNCH		DINNER		BEDTIME	
Sunday	BEFORE	AFTER	BEFORE	AFTER	BEFORE	AFTER	BEFORE	AFTER
BLOOD SUGAR								
BLOOD PRESSURE								

NOTES: _____
_____
_____
_____

Month: _____ **Week Commencing:** _____

Date __/__/__	BREAKFAST		LUNCH		DINNER		BEDTIME	
Monday	BEFORE	AFTER	BEFORE	AFTER	BEFORE	AFTER	BEFORE	AFTER
BLOOD SUGAR								
BLOOD PRESSURE								

Date __/__/__	BREAKFAST		LUNCH		DINNER		BEDTIME	
Tuesday	BEFORE	AFTER	BEFORE	AFTER	BEFORE	AFTER	BEFORE	AFTER
BLOOD SUGAR								
BLOOD PRESSURE								

Date __/__/__	BREAKFAST		LUNCH		DINNER		BEDTIME	
Wednesday	BEFORE	AFTER	BEFORE	AFTER	BEFORE	AFTER	BEFORE	AFTER
BLOOD SUGAR								
BLOOD PRESSURE								

Date __/__/__	BREAKFAST		LUNCH		DINNER		BEDTIME	
Thursday	BEFORE	AFTER	BEFORE	AFTER	BEFORE	AFTER	BEFORE	AFTER
BLOOD SUGAR								
BLOOD PRESSURE								

Date __/__/__	BREAKFAST		LUNCH		DINNER		BEDTIME	
Friday	BEFORE	AFTER	BEFORE	AFTER	BEFORE	AFTER	BEFORE	AFTER
BLOOD SUGAR								
BLOOD PRESSURE								

Date __/__/__	BREAKFAST		LUNCH		DINNER		BEDTIME	
Saturday	BEFORE	AFTER	BEFORE	AFTER	BEFORE	AFTER	BEFORE	AFTER
BLOOD SUGAR								
BLOOD PRESSURE								

Date __/__/__	BREAKFAST		LUNCH		DINNER		BEDTIME	
Sunday	BEFORE	AFTER	BEFORE	AFTER	BEFORE	AFTER	BEFORE	AFTER
BLOOD SUGAR								
BLOOD PRESSURE								

NOTES: _____
_____
_____
_____

Month: _____ **Week Commencing:** _____

Date __/__/__	BREAKFAST		LUNCH		DINNER		BEDTIME	
Monday	BEFORE	AFTER	BEFORE	AFTER	BEFORE	AFTER	BEFORE	AFTER
BLOOD SUGAR								
BLOOD PRESSURE								
Date __/__/__	BREAKFAST		LUNCH		DINNER		BEDTIME	
Tuesday	BEFORE	AFTER	BEFORE	AFTER	BEFORE	AFTER	BEFORE	AFTER
BLOOD SUGAR								
BLOOD PRESSURE								
Date __/__/__	BREAKFAST		LUNCH		DINNER		BEDTIME	
Wednesday	BEFORE	AFTER	BEFORE	AFTER	BEFORE	AFTER	BEFORE	AFTER
BLOOD SUGAR								
BLOOD PRESSURE								
Date __/__/__	BREAKFAST		LUNCH		DINNER		BEDTIME	
Thursday	BEFORE	AFTER	BEFORE	AFTER	BEFORE	AFTER	BEFORE	AFTER
BLOOD SUGAR								
BLOOD PRESSURE								
Date __/__/__	BREAKFAST		LUNCH		DINNER		BEDTIME	
Friday	BEFORE	AFTER	BEFORE	AFTER	BEFORE	AFTER	BEFORE	AFTER
BLOOD SUGAR								
BLOOD PRESSURE								
Date __/__/__	BREAKFAST		LUNCH		DINNER		BEDTIME	
Saturday	BEFORE	AFTER	BEFORE	AFTER	BEFORE	AFTER	BEFORE	AFTER
BLOOD SUGAR								
BLOOD PRESSURE								
Date __/__/__	BREAKFAST		LUNCH		DINNER		BEDTIME	
Sunday	BEFORE	AFTER	BEFORE	AFTER	BEFORE	AFTER	BEFORE	AFTER
BLOOD SUGAR								
BLOOD PRESSURE								

NOTES: _____

_____

_____

_____

Month: _____ **Week Commencing:** _____

Date __/__/__	BREAKFAST		LUNCH		DINNER		BEDTIME	
Monday	BEFORE	AFTER	BEFORE	AFTER	BEFORE	AFTER	BEFORE	AFTER
BLOOD SUGAR								
BLOOD PRESSURE								
Date __/__/__	BREAKFAST		LUNCH		DINNER		BEDTIME	
Tuesday	BEFORE	AFTER	BEFORE	AFTER	BEFORE	AFTER	BEFORE	AFTER
BLOOD SUGAR								
BLOOD PRESSURE								
Date __/__/__	BREAKFAST		LUNCH		DINNER		BEDTIME	
Wednesday	BEFORE	AFTER	BEFORE	AFTER	BEFORE	AFTER	BEFORE	AFTER
BLOOD SUGAR								
BLOOD PRESSURE								
Date __/__/__	BREAKFAST		LUNCH		DINNER		BEDTIME	
Thursday	BEFORE	AFTER	BEFORE	AFTER	BEFORE	AFTER	BEFORE	AFTER
BLOOD SUGAR								
BLOOD PRESSURE								
Date __/__/__	BREAKFAST		LUNCH		DINNER		BEDTIME	
Friday	BEFORE	AFTER	BEFORE	AFTER	BEFORE	AFTER	BEFORE	AFTER
BLOOD SUGAR								
BLOOD PRESSURE								
Date __/__/__	BREAKFAST		LUNCH		DINNER		BEDTIME	
Saturday	BEFORE	AFTER	BEFORE	AFTER	BEFORE	AFTER	BEFORE	AFTER
BLOOD SUGAR								
BLOOD PRESSURE								
Date __/__/__	BREAKFAST		LUNCH		DINNER		BEDTIME	
Sunday	BEFORE	AFTER	BEFORE	AFTER	BEFORE	AFTER	BEFORE	AFTER
BLOOD SUGAR								
BLOOD PRESSURE								

NOTES: _____

_____

_____

_____

Month: _____ **Week Commencing:** _____

Date __/__/__	BREAKFAST		LUNCH		DINNER		BEDTIME	
Monday	BEFORE	AFTER	BEFORE	AFTER	BEFORE	AFTER	BEFORE	AFTER
BLOOD SUGAR								
BLOOD PRESSURE								

Date __/__/__	BREAKFAST		LUNCH		DINNER		BEDTIME	
Tuesday	BEFORE	AFTER	BEFORE	AFTER	BEFORE	AFTER	BEFORE	AFTER
BLOOD SUGAR								
BLOOD PRESSURE								

Date __/__/__	BREAKFAST		LUNCH		DINNER		BEDTIME	
Wednesday	BEFORE	AFTER	BEFORE	AFTER	BEFORE	AFTER	BEFORE	AFTER
BLOOD SUGAR								
BLOOD PRESSURE								

Date __/__/__	BREAKFAST		LUNCH		DINNER		BEDTIME	
Thursday	BEFORE	AFTER	BEFORE	AFTER	BEFORE	AFTER	BEFORE	AFTER
BLOOD SUGAR								
BLOOD PRESSURE								

Date __/__/__	BREAKFAST		LUNCH		DINNER		BEDTIME	
Friday	BEFORE	AFTER	BEFORE	AFTER	BEFORE	AFTER	BEFORE	AFTER
BLOOD SUGAR								
BLOOD PRESSURE								

Date __/__/__	BREAKFAST		LUNCH		DINNER		BEDTIME	
Saturday	BEFORE	AFTER	BEFORE	AFTER	BEFORE	AFTER	BEFORE	AFTER
BLOOD SUGAR								
BLOOD PRESSURE								

Date __/__/__	BREAKFAST		LUNCH		DINNER		BEDTIME	
Sunday	BEFORE	AFTER	BEFORE	AFTER	BEFORE	AFTER	BEFORE	AFTER
BLOOD SUGAR								
BLOOD PRESSURE								

NOTES: _____
_____
_____
_____

Month: _____ **Week Commencing:** _____

Date __/__/__ Monday	BREAKFAST		LUNCH		DINNER		BEDTIME	
	BEFORE	AFTER	BEFORE	AFTER	BEFORE	AFTER	BEFORE	AFTER
BLOOD SUGAR								
BLOOD PRESSURE								

Date __/__/__ Tuesday	BREAKFAST		LUNCH		DINNER		BEDTIME	
	BEFORE	AFTER	BEFORE	AFTER	BEFORE	AFTER	BEFORE	AFTER
BLOOD SUGAR								
BLOOD PRESSURE								

Date __/__/__ Wednesday	BREAKFAST		LUNCH		DINNER		BEDTIME	
	BEFORE	AFTER	BEFORE	AFTER	BEFORE	AFTER	BEFORE	AFTER
BLOOD SUGAR								
BLOOD PRESSURE								

Date __/__/__ Thursday	BREAKFAST		LUNCH		DINNER		BEDTIME	
	BEFORE	AFTER	BEFORE	AFTER	BEFORE	AFTER	BEFORE	AFTER
BLOOD SUGAR								
BLOOD PRESSURE								

Date __/__/__ Friday	BREAKFAST		LUNCH		DINNER		BEDTIME	
	BEFORE	AFTER	BEFORE	AFTER	BEFORE	AFTER	BEFORE	AFTER
BLOOD SUGAR								
BLOOD PRESSURE								

Date __/__/__ Saturday	BREAKFAST		LUNCH		DINNER		BEDTIME	
	BEFORE	AFTER	BEFORE	AFTER	BEFORE	AFTER	BEFORE	AFTER
BLOOD SUGAR								
BLOOD PRESSURE								

Date __/__/__ Sunday	BREAKFAST		LUNCH		DINNER		BEDTIME	
	BEFORE	AFTER	BEFORE	AFTER	BEFORE	AFTER	BEFORE	AFTER
BLOOD SUGAR								
BLOOD PRESSURE								

NOTES: _____
_____
_____
_____

Month: _____ **Week Commencing:** _____

Date __/__/__ Monday	BREAKFAST		LUNCH		DINNER		BEDTIME	
	BEFORE	AFTER	BEFORE	AFTER	BEFORE	AFTER	BEFORE	AFTER
BLOOD SUGAR								
BLOOD PRESSURE								

Date __/__/__ Tuesday	BREAKFAST		LUNCH		DINNER		BEDTIME	
	BEFORE	AFTER	BEFORE	AFTER	BEFORE	AFTER	BEFORE	AFTER
BLOOD SUGAR								
BLOOD PRESSURE								

Date __/__/__ Wednesday	BREAKFAST		LUNCH		DINNER		BEDTIME	
	BEFORE	AFTER	BEFORE	AFTER	BEFORE	AFTER	BEFORE	AFTER
BLOOD SUGAR								
BLOOD PRESSURE								

Date __/__/__ Thursday	BREAKFAST		LUNCH		DINNER		BEDTIME	
	BEFORE	AFTER	BEFORE	AFTER	BEFORE	AFTER	BEFORE	AFTER
BLOOD SUGAR								
BLOOD PRESSURE								

Date __/__/__ Friday	BREAKFAST		LUNCH		DINNER		BEDTIME	
	BEFORE	AFTER	BEFORE	AFTER	BEFORE	AFTER	BEFORE	AFTER
BLOOD SUGAR								
BLOOD PRESSURE								

Date __/__/__ Saturday	BREAKFAST		LUNCH		DINNER		BEDTIME	
	BEFORE	AFTER	BEFORE	AFTER	BEFORE	AFTER	BEFORE	AFTER
BLOOD SUGAR								
BLOOD PRESSURE								

Date __/__/__ Sunday	BREAKFAST		LUNCH		DINNER		BEDTIME	
	BEFORE	AFTER	BEFORE	AFTER	BEFORE	AFTER	BEFORE	AFTER
BLOOD SUGAR								
BLOOD PRESSURE								

NOTES: _____
_____
_____
_____

Month: _____ **Week Commencing:** _____

Date __/__/__	BREAKFAST		LUNCH		DINNER		BEDTIME	
Monday	BEFORE	AFTER	BEFORE	AFTER	BEFORE	AFTER	BEFORE	AFTER
BLOOD SUGAR								
BLOOD PRESSURE								
Date __/__/__	BREAKFAST		LUNCH		DINNER		BEDTIME	
Tuesday	BEFORE	AFTER	BEFORE	AFTER	BEFORE	AFTER	BEFORE	AFTER
BLOOD SUGAR								
BLOOD PRESSURE								
Date __/__/__	BREAKFAST		LUNCH		DINNER		BEDTIME	
Wednesday	BEFORE	AFTER	BEFORE	AFTER	BEFORE	AFTER	BEFORE	AFTER
BLOOD SUGAR								
BLOOD PRESSURE								
Date __/__/__	BREAKFAST		LUNCH		DINNER		BEDTIME	
Thursday	BEFORE	AFTER	BEFORE	AFTER	BEFORE	AFTER	BEFORE	AFTER
BLOOD SUGAR								
BLOOD PRESSURE								
Date __/__/__	BREAKFAST		LUNCH		DINNER		BEDTIME	
Friday	BEFORE	AFTER	BEFORE	AFTER	BEFORE	AFTER	BEFORE	AFTER
BLOOD SUGAR								
BLOOD PRESSURE								
Date __/__/__	BREAKFAST		LUNCH		DINNER		BEDTIME	
Saturday	BEFORE	AFTER	BEFORE	AFTER	BEFORE	AFTER	BEFORE	AFTER
BLOOD SUGAR								
BLOOD PRESSURE								
Date __/__/__	BREAKFAST		LUNCH		DINNER		BEDTIME	
Sunday	BEFORE	AFTER	BEFORE	AFTER	BEFORE	AFTER	BEFORE	AFTER
BLOOD SUGAR								
BLOOD PRESSURE								

NOTES: _____
_____
_____
_____

Month: _____ Week Commencing: _____

Date __/__/__	BREAKFAST		LUNCH		DINNER		BEDTIME	
Monday	BEFORE	AFTER	BEFORE	AFTER	BEFORE	AFTER	BEFORE	AFTER
BLOOD SUGAR								
BLOOD PRESSURE								
Date __/__/__	BREAKFAST		LUNCH		DINNER		BEDTIME	
Tuesday	BEFORE	AFTER	BEFORE	AFTER	BEFORE	AFTER	BEFORE	AFTER
BLOOD SUGAR								
BLOOD PRESSURE								
Date __/__/__	BREAKFAST		LUNCH		DINNER		BEDTIME	
Wednesday	BEFORE	AFTER	BEFORE	AFTER	BEFORE	AFTER	BEFORE	AFTER
BLOOD SUGAR								
BLOOD PRESSURE								
Date __/__/__	BREAKFAST		LUNCH		DINNER		BEDTIME	
Thursday	BEFORE	AFTER	BEFORE	AFTER	BEFORE	AFTER	BEFORE	AFTER
BLOOD SUGAR								
BLOOD PRESSURE								
Date __/__/__	BREAKFAST		LUNCH		DINNER		BEDTIME	
Friday	BEFORE	AFTER	BEFORE	AFTER	BEFORE	AFTER	BEFORE	AFTER
BLOOD SUGAR								
BLOOD PRESSURE								
Date __/__/__	BREAKFAST		LUNCH		DINNER		BEDTIME	
Saturday	BEFORE	AFTER	BEFORE	AFTER	BEFORE	AFTER	BEFORE	AFTER
BLOOD SUGAR								
BLOOD PRESSURE								
Date __/__/__	BREAKFAST		LUNCH		DINNER		BEDTIME	
Sunday	BEFORE	AFTER	BEFORE	AFTER	BEFORE	AFTER	BEFORE	AFTER
BLOOD SUGAR								
BLOOD PRESSURE								

NOTES: _____
_____
_____
_____

Month: _____ **Week Commencing:** _____

Date __/__/__	BREAKFAST		LUNCH		DINNER		BEDTIME	
Monday	BEFORE	AFTER	BEFORE	AFTER	BEFORE	AFTER	BEFORE	AFTER
BLOOD SUGAR								
BLOOD PRESSURE								
Date __/__/__	BREAKFAST		LUNCH		DINNER		BEDTIME	
Tuesday	BEFORE	AFTER	BEFORE	AFTER	BEFORE	AFTER	BEFORE	AFTER
BLOOD SUGAR								
BLOOD PRESSURE								
Date __/__/__	BREAKFAST		LUNCH		DINNER		BEDTIME	
Wednesday	BEFORE	AFTER	BEFORE	AFTER	BEFORE	AFTER	BEFORE	AFTER
BLOOD SUGAR								
BLOOD PRESSURE								
Date __/__/__	BREAKFAST		LUNCH		DINNER		BEDTIME	
Thursday	BEFORE	AFTER	BEFORE	AFTER	BEFORE	AFTER	BEFORE	AFTER
BLOOD SUGAR								
BLOOD PRESSURE								
Date __/__/__	BREAKFAST		LUNCH		DINNER		BEDTIME	
Friday	BEFORE	AFTER	BEFORE	AFTER	BEFORE	AFTER	BEFORE	AFTER
BLOOD SUGAR								
BLOOD PRESSURE								
Date __/__/__	BREAKFAST		LUNCH		DINNER		BEDTIME	
Saturday	BEFORE	AFTER	BEFORE	AFTER	BEFORE	AFTER	BEFORE	AFTER
BLOOD SUGAR								
BLOOD PRESSURE								
Date __/__/__	BREAKFAST		LUNCH		DINNER		BEDTIME	
Sunday	BEFORE	AFTER	BEFORE	AFTER	BEFORE	AFTER	BEFORE	AFTER
BLOOD SUGAR								
BLOOD PRESSURE								

NOTES: _____
_____
_____
_____

Month: _____ **Week Commencing:** _____

Date __/__/__	BREAKFAST		LUNCH		DINNER		BEDTIME	
Monday	BEFORE	AFTER	BEFORE	AFTER	BEFORE	AFTER	BEFORE	AFTER
BLOOD SUGAR								
BLOOD PRESSURE								
Date __/__/__	BREAKFAST		LUNCH		DINNER		BEDTIME	
Tuesday	BEFORE	AFTER	BEFORE	AFTER	BEFORE	AFTER	BEFORE	AFTER
BLOOD SUGAR								
BLOOD PRESSURE								
Date __/__/__	BREAKFAST		LUNCH		DINNER		BEDTIME	
Wednesday	BEFORE	AFTER	BEFORE	AFTER	BEFORE	AFTER	BEFORE	AFTER
BLOOD SUGAR								
BLOOD PRESSURE								
Date __/__/__	BREAKFAST		LUNCH		DINNER		BEDTIME	
Thursday	BEFORE	AFTER	BEFORE	AFTER	BEFORE	AFTER	BEFORE	AFTER
BLOOD SUGAR								
BLOOD PRESSURE								
Date __/__/__	BREAKFAST		LUNCH		DINNER		BEDTIME	
Friday	BEFORE	AFTER	BEFORE	AFTER	BEFORE	AFTER	BEFORE	AFTER
BLOOD SUGAR								
BLOOD PRESSURE								
Date __/__/__	BREAKFAST		LUNCH		DINNER		BEDTIME	
Saturday	BEFORE	AFTER	BEFORE	AFTER	BEFORE	AFTER	BEFORE	AFTER
BLOOD SUGAR								
BLOOD PRESSURE								
Date __/__/__	BREAKFAST		LUNCH		DINNER		BEDTIME	
Sunday	BEFORE	AFTER	BEFORE	AFTER	BEFORE	AFTER	BEFORE	AFTER
BLOOD SUGAR								
BLOOD PRESSURE								

NOTES: _____
_____
_____
_____

Month: _____ **Week Commencing:** _____

Date __/__/__	BREAKFAST		LUNCH		DINNER		BEDTIME	
Monday	BEFORE	AFTER	BEFORE	AFTER	BEFORE	AFTER	BEFORE	AFTER
BLOOD SUGAR								
BLOOD PRESSURE								
Date __/__/__	BREAKFAST		LUNCH		DINNER		BEDTIME	
Tuesday	BEFORE	AFTER	BEFORE	AFTER	BEFORE	AFTER	BEFORE	AFTER
BLOOD SUGAR								
BLOOD PRESSURE								
Date __/__/__	BREAKFAST		LUNCH		DINNER		BEDTIME	
Wednesday	BEFORE	AFTER	BEFORE	AFTER	BEFORE	AFTER	BEFORE	AFTER
BLOOD SUGAR								
BLOOD PRESSURE								
Date __/__/__	BREAKFAST		LUNCH		DINNER		BEDTIME	
Thursday	BEFORE	AFTER	BEFORE	AFTER	BEFORE	AFTER	BEFORE	AFTER
BLOOD SUGAR								
BLOOD PRESSURE								
Date __/__/__	BREAKFAST		LUNCH		DINNER		BEDTIME	
Friday	BEFORE	AFTER	BEFORE	AFTER	BEFORE	AFTER	BEFORE	AFTER
BLOOD SUGAR								
BLOOD PRESSURE								
Date __/__/__	BREAKFAST		LUNCH		DINNER		BEDTIME	
Saturday	BEFORE	AFTER	BEFORE	AFTER	BEFORE	AFTER	BEFORE	AFTER
BLOOD SUGAR								
BLOOD PRESSURE								
Date __/__/__	BREAKFAST		LUNCH		DINNER		BEDTIME	
Sunday	BEFORE	AFTER	BEFORE	AFTER	BEFORE	AFTER	BEFORE	AFTER
BLOOD SUGAR								
BLOOD PRESSURE								

NOTES: _____
_____
_____
_____

Month: _____ **Week Commencing:** _____

Date __/__/__	BREAKFAST		LUNCH		DINNER		BEDTIME	
Monday	BEFORE	AFTER	BEFORE	AFTER	BEFORE	AFTER	BEFORE	AFTER
BLOOD SUGAR								
BLOOD PRESSURE								
Date __/__/__	BREAKFAST		LUNCH		DINNER		BEDTIME	
Tuesday	BEFORE	AFTER	BEFORE	AFTER	BEFORE	AFTER	BEFORE	AFTER
BLOOD SUGAR								
BLOOD PRESSURE								
Date __/__/__	BREAKFAST		LUNCH		DINNER		BEDTIME	
Wednesday	BEFORE	AFTER	BEFORE	AFTER	BEFORE	AFTER	BEFORE	AFTER
BLOOD SUGAR								
BLOOD PRESSURE								
Date __/__/__	BREAKFAST		LUNCH		DINNER		BEDTIME	
Thursday	BEFORE	AFTER	BEFORE	AFTER	BEFORE	AFTER	BEFORE	AFTER
BLOOD SUGAR								
BLOOD PRESSURE								
Date __/__/__	BREAKFAST		LUNCH		DINNER		BEDTIME	
Friday	BEFORE	AFTER	BEFORE	AFTER	BEFORE	AFTER	BEFORE	AFTER
BLOOD SUGAR								
BLOOD PRESSURE								
Date __/__/__	BREAKFAST		LUNCH		DINNER		BEDTIME	
Saturday	BEFORE	AFTER	BEFORE	AFTER	BEFORE	AFTER	BEFORE	AFTER
BLOOD SUGAR								
BLOOD PRESSURE								
Date __/__/__	BREAKFAST		LUNCH		DINNER		BEDTIME	
Sunday	BEFORE	AFTER	BEFORE	AFTER	BEFORE	AFTER	BEFORE	AFTER
BLOOD SUGAR								
BLOOD PRESSURE								

NOTES: _____

_____

_____

Month: _____ Week Commencing: _____

Date __/__/__	BREAKFAST		LUNCH		DINNER		BEDTIME	
Monday	BEFORE	AFTER	BEFORE	AFTER	BEFORE	AFTER	BEFORE	AFTER
BLOOD SUGAR								
BLOOD PRESSURE								
Date __/__/__	BREAKFAST		LUNCH		DINNER		BEDTIME	
Tuesday	BEFORE	AFTER	BEFORE	AFTER	BEFORE	AFTER	BEFORE	AFTER
BLOOD SUGAR								
BLOOD PRESSURE								
Date __/__/__	BREAKFAST		LUNCH		DINNER		BEDTIME	
Wednesday	BEFORE	AFTER	BEFORE	AFTER	BEFORE	AFTER	BEFORE	AFTER
BLOOD SUGAR								
BLOOD PRESSURE								
Date __/__/__	BREAKFAST		LUNCH		DINNER		BEDTIME	
Thursday	BEFORE	AFTER	BEFORE	AFTER	BEFORE	AFTER	BEFORE	AFTER
BLOOD SUGAR								
BLOOD PRESSURE								
Date __/__/__	BREAKFAST		LUNCH		DINNER		BEDTIME	
Friday	BEFORE	AFTER	BEFORE	AFTER	BEFORE	AFTER	BEFORE	AFTER
BLOOD SUGAR								
BLOOD PRESSURE								
Date __/__/__	BREAKFAST		LUNCH		DINNER		BEDTIME	
Saturday	BEFORE	AFTER	BEFORE	AFTER	BEFORE	AFTER	BEFORE	AFTER
BLOOD SUGAR								
BLOOD PRESSURE								
Date __/__/__	BREAKFAST		LUNCH		DINNER		BEDTIME	
Sunday	BEFORE	AFTER	BEFORE	AFTER	BEFORE	AFTER	BEFORE	AFTER
BLOOD SUGAR								
BLOOD PRESSURE								

NOTES: _____
_____
_____
_____

Month: _____ **Week Commencing:** _____

Date __/__/__	BREAKFAST		LUNCH		DINNER		BEDTIME	
Monday	BEFORE	AFTER	BEFORE	AFTER	BEFORE	AFTER	BEFORE	AFTER
BLOOD SUGAR								
BLOOD PRESSURE								
Date __/__/__	BREAKFAST		LUNCH		DINNER		BEDTIME	
Tuesday	BEFORE	AFTER	BEFORE	AFTER	BEFORE	AFTER	BEFORE	AFTER
BLOOD SUGAR								
BLOOD PRESSURE								
Date __/__/__	BREAKFAST		LUNCH		DINNER		BEDTIME	
Wednesday	BEFORE	AFTER	BEFORE	AFTER	BEFORE	AFTER	BEFORE	AFTER
BLOOD SUGAR								
BLOOD PRESSURE								
Date __/__/__	BREAKFAST		LUNCH		DINNER		BEDTIME	
Thursday	BEFORE	AFTER	BEFORE	AFTER	BEFORE	AFTER	BEFORE	AFTER
BLOOD SUGAR								
BLOOD PRESSURE								
Date __/__/__	BREAKFAST		LUNCH		DINNER		BEDTIME	
Friday	BEFORE	AFTER	BEFORE	AFTER	BEFORE	AFTER	BEFORE	AFTER
BLOOD SUGAR								
BLOOD PRESSURE								
Date __/__/__	BREAKFAST		LUNCH		DINNER		BEDTIME	
Saturday	BEFORE	AFTER	BEFORE	AFTER	BEFORE	AFTER	BEFORE	AFTER
BLOOD SUGAR								
BLOOD PRESSURE								
Date __/__/__	BREAKFAST		LUNCH		DINNER		BEDTIME	
Sunday	BEFORE	AFTER	BEFORE	AFTER	BEFORE	AFTER	BEFORE	AFTER
BLOOD SUGAR								
BLOOD PRESSURE								

NOTES: _____
_____
_____
_____

Month: _____ **Week Commencing:** _____

Date ___/___/___	BREAKFAST		LUNCH		DINNER		BEDTIME	
Monday	BEFORE	AFTER	BEFORE	AFTER	BEFORE	AFTER	BEFORE	AFTER
BLOOD SUGAR								
BLOOD PRESSURE								
Date ___/___/___	BREAKFAST		LUNCH		DINNER		BEDTIME	
Tuesday	BEFORE	AFTER	BEFORE	AFTER	BEFORE	AFTER	BEFORE	AFTER
BLOOD SUGAR								
BLOOD PRESSURE								
Date ___/___/___	BREAKFAST		LUNCH		DINNER		BEDTIME	
Wednesday	BEFORE	AFTER	BEFORE	AFTER	BEFORE	AFTER	BEFORE	AFTER
BLOOD SUGAR								
BLOOD PRESSURE								
Date ___/___/___	BREAKFAST		LUNCH		DINNER		BEDTIME	
Thursday	BEFORE	AFTER	BEFORE	AFTER	BEFORE	AFTER	BEFORE	AFTER
BLOOD SUGAR								
BLOOD PRESSURE								
Date ___/___/___	BREAKFAST		LUNCH		DINNER		BEDTIME	
Friday	BEFORE	AFTER	BEFORE	AFTER	BEFORE	AFTER	BEFORE	AFTER
BLOOD SUGAR								
BLOOD PRESSURE								
Date ___/___/___	BREAKFAST		LUNCH		DINNER		BEDTIME	
Saturday	BEFORE	AFTER	BEFORE	AFTER	BEFORE	AFTER	BEFORE	AFTER
BLOOD SUGAR								
BLOOD PRESSURE								
Date ___/___/___	BREAKFAST		LUNCH		DINNER		BEDTIME	
Sunday	BEFORE	AFTER	BEFORE	AFTER	BEFORE	AFTER	BEFORE	AFTER
BLOOD SUGAR								
BLOOD PRESSURE								

NOTES: _____
_____
_____
_____

Month: _____ **Week Commencing:** _____

Date __/__/__	BREAKFAST		LUNCH		DINNER		BEDTIME	
Monday	BEFORE	AFTER	BEFORE	AFTER	BEFORE	AFTER	BEFORE	AFTER
BLOOD SUGAR								
BLOOD PRESSURE								
Date __/__/__	BREAKFAST		LUNCH		DINNER		BEDTIME	
Tuesday	BEFORE	AFTER	BEFORE	AFTER	BEFORE	AFTER	BEFORE	AFTER
BLOOD SUGAR								
BLOOD PRESSURE								
Date __/__/__	BREAKFAST		LUNCH		DINNER		BEDTIME	
Wednesday	BEFORE	AFTER	BEFORE	AFTER	BEFORE	AFTER	BEFORE	AFTER
BLOOD SUGAR								
BLOOD PRESSURE								
Date __/__/__	BREAKFAST		LUNCH		DINNER		BEDTIME	
Thursday	BEFORE	AFTER	BEFORE	AFTER	BEFORE	AFTER	BEFORE	AFTER
BLOOD SUGAR								
BLOOD PRESSURE								
Date __/__/__	BREAKFAST		LUNCH		DINNER		BEDTIME	
Friday	BEFORE	AFTER	BEFORE	AFTER	BEFORE	AFTER	BEFORE	AFTER
BLOOD SUGAR								
BLOOD PRESSURE								
Date __/__/__	BREAKFAST		LUNCH		DINNER		BEDTIME	
Saturday	BEFORE	AFTER	BEFORE	AFTER	BEFORE	AFTER	BEFORE	AFTER
BLOOD SUGAR								
BLOOD PRESSURE								
Date __/__/__	BREAKFAST		LUNCH		DINNER		BEDTIME	
Sunday	BEFORE	AFTER	BEFORE	AFTER	BEFORE	AFTER	BEFORE	AFTER
BLOOD SUGAR								
BLOOD PRESSURE								

NOTES: _____
_____
_____
_____

Month: _____ Week Commencing: _____

Date __/__/__	BREAKFAST		LUNCH		DINNER		BEDTIME	
Monday	BEFORE	AFTER	BEFORE	AFTER	BEFORE	AFTER	BEFORE	AFTER
BLOOD SUGAR								
BLOOD PRESSURE								
Date __/__/__	BREAKFAST		LUNCH		DINNER		BEDTIME	
Tuesday	BEFORE	AFTER	BEFORE	AFTER	BEFORE	AFTER	BEFORE	AFTER
BLOOD SUGAR								
BLOOD PRESSURE								
Date __/__/__	BREAKFAST		LUNCH		DINNER		BEDTIME	
Wednesday	BEFORE	AFTER	BEFORE	AFTER	BEFORE	AFTER	BEFORE	AFTER
BLOOD SUGAR								
BLOOD PRESSURE								
Date __/__/__	BREAKFAST		LUNCH		DINNER		BEDTIME	
Thursday	BEFORE	AFTER	BEFORE	AFTER	BEFORE	AFTER	BEFORE	AFTER
BLOOD SUGAR								
BLOOD PRESSURE								
Date __/__/__	BREAKFAST		LUNCH		DINNER		BEDTIME	
Friday	BEFORE	AFTER	BEFORE	AFTER	BEFORE	AFTER	BEFORE	AFTER
BLOOD SUGAR								
BLOOD PRESSURE								
Date __/__/__	BREAKFAST		LUNCH		DINNER		BEDTIME	
Saturday	BEFORE	AFTER	BEFORE	AFTER	BEFORE	AFTER	BEFORE	AFTER
BLOOD SUGAR								
BLOOD PRESSURE								
Date __/__/__	BREAKFAST		LUNCH		DINNER		BEDTIME	
Sunday	BEFORE	AFTER	BEFORE	AFTER	BEFORE	AFTER	BEFORE	AFTER
BLOOD SUGAR								
BLOOD PRESSURE								

NOTES: _____
_____
_____
_____

Month: _____ **Week Commencing:** _____

Date __/__/__	BREAKFAST		LUNCH		DINNER		BEDTIME	
Monday	BEFORE	AFTER	BEFORE	AFTER	BEFORE	AFTER	BEFORE	AFTER
BLOOD SUGAR								
BLOOD PRESSURE								
Date __/__/__	BREAKFAST		LUNCH		DINNER		BEDTIME	
Tuesday	BEFORE	AFTER	BEFORE	AFTER	BEFORE	AFTER	BEFORE	AFTER
BLOOD SUGAR								
BLOOD PRESSURE								
Date __/__/__	BREAKFAST		LUNCH		DINNER		BEDTIME	
Wednesday	BEFORE	AFTER	BEFORE	AFTER	BEFORE	AFTER	BEFORE	AFTER
BLOOD SUGAR								
BLOOD PRESSURE								
Date __/__/__	BREAKFAST		LUNCH		DINNER		BEDTIME	
Thursday	BEFORE	AFTER	BEFORE	AFTER	BEFORE	AFTER	BEFORE	AFTER
BLOOD SUGAR								
BLOOD PRESSURE								
Date __/__/__	BREAKFAST		LUNCH		DINNER		BEDTIME	
Friday	BEFORE	AFTER	BEFORE	AFTER	BEFORE	AFTER	BEFORE	AFTER
BLOOD SUGAR								
BLOOD PRESSURE								
Date __/__/__	BREAKFAST		LUNCH		DINNER		BEDTIME	
Saturday	BEFORE	AFTER	BEFORE	AFTER	BEFORE	AFTER	BEFORE	AFTER
BLOOD SUGAR								
BLOOD PRESSURE								
Date __/__/__	BREAKFAST		LUNCH		DINNER		BEDTIME	
Sunday	BEFORE	AFTER	BEFORE	AFTER	BEFORE	AFTER	BEFORE	AFTER
BLOOD SUGAR								
BLOOD PRESSURE								

NOTES: _____

_____

_____

Month: _____ **Week Commencing:** _____

Date __/__/__	BREAKFAST		LUNCH		DINNER		BEDTIME	
Monday	BEFORE	AFTER	BEFORE	AFTER	BEFORE	AFTER	BEFORE	AFTER
BLOOD SUGAR								
BLOOD PRESSURE								
Date __/__/__	BREAKFAST		LUNCH		DINNER		BEDTIME	
Tuesday	BEFORE	AFTER	BEFORE	AFTER	BEFORE	AFTER	BEFORE	AFTER
BLOOD SUGAR								
BLOOD PRESSURE								
Date __/__/__	BREAKFAST		LUNCH		DINNER		BEDTIME	
Wednesday	BEFORE	AFTER	BEFORE	AFTER	BEFORE	AFTER	BEFORE	AFTER
BLOOD SUGAR								
BLOOD PRESSURE								
Date __/__/__	BREAKFAST		LUNCH		DINNER		BEDTIME	
Thursday	BEFORE	AFTER	BEFORE	AFTER	BEFORE	AFTER	BEFORE	AFTER
BLOOD SUGAR								
BLOOD PRESSURE								
Date __/__/__	BREAKFAST		LUNCH		DINNER		BEDTIME	
Friday	BEFORE	AFTER	BEFORE	AFTER	BEFORE	AFTER	BEFORE	AFTER
BLOOD SUGAR								
BLOOD PRESSURE								
Date __/__/__	BREAKFAST		LUNCH		DINNER		BEDTIME	
Saturday	BEFORE	AFTER	BEFORE	AFTER	BEFORE	AFTER	BEFORE	AFTER
BLOOD SUGAR								
BLOOD PRESSURE								
Date __/__/__	BREAKFAST		LUNCH		DINNER		BEDTIME	
Sunday	BEFORE	AFTER	BEFORE	AFTER	BEFORE	AFTER	BEFORE	AFTER
BLOOD SUGAR								
BLOOD PRESSURE								

NOTES: _____

_____

_____

_____

Month: _____ **Week Commencing:** _____

Date __/__/__	BREAKFAST		LUNCH		DINNER		BEDTIME	
Monday	BEFORE	AFTER	BEFORE	AFTER	BEFORE	AFTER	BEFORE	AFTER
BLOOD SUGAR								
BLOOD PRESSURE								
Date __/__/__	BREAKFAST		LUNCH		DINNER		BEDTIME	
Tuesday	BEFORE	AFTER	BEFORE	AFTER	BEFORE	AFTER	BEFORE	AFTER
BLOOD SUGAR								
BLOOD PRESSURE								
Date __/__/__	BREAKFAST		LUNCH		DINNER		BEDTIME	
Wednesday	BEFORE	AFTER	BEFORE	AFTER	BEFORE	AFTER	BEFORE	AFTER
BLOOD SUGAR								
BLOOD PRESSURE								
Date __/__/__	BREAKFAST		LUNCH		DINNER		BEDTIME	
Thursday	BEFORE	AFTER	BEFORE	AFTER	BEFORE	AFTER	BEFORE	AFTER
BLOOD SUGAR								
BLOOD PRESSURE								
Date __/__/__	BREAKFAST		LUNCH		DINNER		BEDTIME	
Friday	BEFORE	AFTER	BEFORE	AFTER	BEFORE	AFTER	BEFORE	AFTER
BLOOD SUGAR								
BLOOD PRESSURE								
Date __/__/__	BREAKFAST		LUNCH		DINNER		BEDTIME	
Saturday	BEFORE	AFTER	BEFORE	AFTER	BEFORE	AFTER	BEFORE	AFTER
BLOOD SUGAR								
BLOOD PRESSURE								
Date __/__/__	BREAKFAST		LUNCH		DINNER		BEDTIME	
Sunday	BEFORE	AFTER	BEFORE	AFTER	BEFORE	AFTER	BEFORE	AFTER
BLOOD SUGAR								
BLOOD PRESSURE								

NOTES: _____
_____
_____
_____

Month: _____ **Week Commencing:** _____

Date __/__/__	BREAKFAST		LUNCH		DINNER		BEDTIME	
Monday	BEFORE	AFTER	BEFORE	AFTER	BEFORE	AFTER	BEFORE	AFTER
BLOOD SUGAR								
BLOOD PRESSURE								

Date __/__/__	BREAKFAST		LUNCH		DINNER		BEDTIME	
Tuesday	BEFORE	AFTER	BEFORE	AFTER	BEFORE	AFTER	BEFORE	AFTER
BLOOD SUGAR								
BLOOD PRESSURE								

Date __/__/__	BREAKFAST		LUNCH		DINNER		BEDTIME	
Wednesday	BEFORE	AFTER	BEFORE	AFTER	BEFORE	AFTER	BEFORE	AFTER
BLOOD SUGAR								
BLOOD PRESSURE								

Date __/__/__	BREAKFAST		LUNCH		DINNER		BEDTIME	
Thursday	BEFORE	AFTER	BEFORE	AFTER	BEFORE	AFTER	BEFORE	AFTER
BLOOD SUGAR								
BLOOD PRESSURE								

Date __/__/__	BREAKFAST		LUNCH		DINNER		BEDTIME	
Friday	BEFORE	AFTER	BEFORE	AFTER	BEFORE	AFTER	BEFORE	AFTER
BLOOD SUGAR								
BLOOD PRESSURE								

Date __/__/__	BREAKFAST		LUNCH		DINNER		BEDTIME	
Saturday	BEFORE	AFTER	BEFORE	AFTER	BEFORE	AFTER	BEFORE	AFTER
BLOOD SUGAR								
BLOOD PRESSURE								

Date __/__/__	BREAKFAST		LUNCH		DINNER		BEDTIME	
Sunday	BEFORE	AFTER	BEFORE	AFTER	BEFORE	AFTER	BEFORE	AFTER
BLOOD SUGAR								
BLOOD PRESSURE								

NOTES: _____
_____
_____
_____

Month: _____ **Week Commencing:** _____

Date __/__/__	BREAKFAST		LUNCH		DINNER		BEDTIME	
Monday	BEFORE	AFTER	BEFORE	AFTER	BEFORE	AFTER	BEFORE	AFTER
BLOOD SUGAR								
BLOOD PRESSURE								
Date __/__/__	BREAKFAST		LUNCH		DINNER		BEDTIME	
Tuesday	BEFORE	AFTER	BEFORE	AFTER	BEFORE	AFTER	BEFORE	AFTER
BLOOD SUGAR								
BLOOD PRESSURE								
Date __/__/__	BREAKFAST		LUNCH		DINNER		BEDTIME	
Wednesday	BEFORE	AFTER	BEFORE	AFTER	BEFORE	AFTER	BEFORE	AFTER
BLOOD SUGAR								
BLOOD PRESSURE								
Date __/__/__	BREAKFAST		LUNCH		DINNER		BEDTIME	
Thursday	BEFORE	AFTER	BEFORE	AFTER	BEFORE	AFTER	BEFORE	AFTER
BLOOD SUGAR								
BLOOD PRESSURE								
Date __/__/__	BREAKFAST		LUNCH		DINNER		BEDTIME	
Friday	BEFORE	AFTER	BEFORE	AFTER	BEFORE	AFTER	BEFORE	AFTER
BLOOD SUGAR								
BLOOD PRESSURE								
Date __/__/__	BREAKFAST		LUNCH		DINNER		BEDTIME	
Saturday	BEFORE	AFTER	BEFORE	AFTER	BEFORE	AFTER	BEFORE	AFTER
BLOOD SUGAR								
BLOOD PRESSURE								
Date __/__/__	BREAKFAST		LUNCH		DINNER		BEDTIME	
Sunday	BEFORE	AFTER	BEFORE	AFTER	BEFORE	AFTER	BEFORE	AFTER
BLOOD SUGAR								
BLOOD PRESSURE								

NOTES: _____

_____

_____

Month: _____ **Week Commencing:** _____

Date __/__/__	BREAKFAST		LUNCH		DINNER		BEDTIME	
Monday	BEFORE	AFTER	BEFORE	AFTER	BEFORE	AFTER	BEFORE	AFTER
BLOOD SUGAR								
BLOOD PRESSURE								
Date __/__/__	BREAKFAST		LUNCH		DINNER		BEDTIME	
Tuesday	BEFORE	AFTER	BEFORE	AFTER	BEFORE	AFTER	BEFORE	AFTER
BLOOD SUGAR								
BLOOD PRESSURE								
Date __/__/__	BREAKFAST		LUNCH		DINNER		BEDTIME	
Wednesday	BEFORE	AFTER	BEFORE	AFTER	BEFORE	AFTER	BEFORE	AFTER
BLOOD SUGAR								
BLOOD PRESSURE								
Date __/__/__	BREAKFAST		LUNCH		DINNER		BEDTIME	
Thursday	BEFORE	AFTER	BEFORE	AFTER	BEFORE	AFTER	BEFORE	AFTER
BLOOD SUGAR								
BLOOD PRESSURE								
Date __/__/__	BREAKFAST		LUNCH		DINNER		BEDTIME	
Friday	BEFORE	AFTER	BEFORE	AFTER	BEFORE	AFTER	BEFORE	AFTER
BLOOD SUGAR								
BLOOD PRESSURE								
Date __/__/__	BREAKFAST		LUNCH		DINNER		BEDTIME	
Saturday	BEFORE	AFTER	BEFORE	AFTER	BEFORE	AFTER	BEFORE	AFTER
BLOOD SUGAR								
BLOOD PRESSURE								
Date __/__/__	BREAKFAST		LUNCH		DINNER		BEDTIME	
Sunday	BEFORE	AFTER	BEFORE	AFTER	BEFORE	AFTER	BEFORE	AFTER
BLOOD SUGAR								
BLOOD PRESSURE								

NOTES: _____

_____

_____

_____

Month: _____ **Week Commencing:** _____

Date __/__/__	BREAKFAST		LUNCH		DINNER		BEDTIME	
Monday	BEFORE	AFTER	BEFORE	AFTER	BEFORE	AFTER	BEFORE	AFTER
BLOOD SUGAR								
BLOOD PRESSURE								
Date __/__/__	BREAKFAST		LUNCH		DINNER		BEDTIME	
Tuesday	BEFORE	AFTER	BEFORE	AFTER	BEFORE	AFTER	BEFORE	AFTER
BLOOD SUGAR								
BLOOD PRESSURE								
Date __/__/__	BREAKFAST		LUNCH		DINNER		BEDTIME	
Wednesday	BEFORE	AFTER	BEFORE	AFTER	BEFORE	AFTER	BEFORE	AFTER
BLOOD SUGAR								
BLOOD PRESSURE								
Date __/__/__	BREAKFAST		LUNCH		DINNER		BEDTIME	
Thursday	BEFORE	AFTER	BEFORE	AFTER	BEFORE	AFTER	BEFORE	AFTER
BLOOD SUGAR								
BLOOD PRESSURE								
Date __/__/__	BREAKFAST		LUNCH		DINNER		BEDTIME	
Friday	BEFORE	AFTER	BEFORE	AFTER	BEFORE	AFTER	BEFORE	AFTER
BLOOD SUGAR								
BLOOD PRESSURE								
Date __/__/__	BREAKFAST		LUNCH		DINNER		BEDTIME	
Saturday	BEFORE	AFTER	BEFORE	AFTER	BEFORE	AFTER	BEFORE	AFTER
BLOOD SUGAR								
BLOOD PRESSURE								
Date __/__/__	BREAKFAST		LUNCH		DINNER		BEDTIME	
Sunday	BEFORE	AFTER	BEFORE	AFTER	BEFORE	AFTER	BEFORE	AFTER
BLOOD SUGAR								
BLOOD PRESSURE								

NOTES: _____
_____
_____
_____

Month: _____ **Week Commencing:** _____

Date __/__/__	BREAKFAST		LUNCH		DINNER		BEDTIME	
Monday	BEFORE	AFTER	BEFORE	AFTER	BEFORE	AFTER	BEFORE	AFTER
BLOOD SUGAR								
BLOOD PRESSURE								
Date __/__/__	BREAKFAST		LUNCH		DINNER		BEDTIME	
Tuesday	BEFORE	AFTER	BEFORE	AFTER	BEFORE	AFTER	BEFORE	AFTER
BLOOD SUGAR								
BLOOD PRESSURE								
Date __/__/__	BREAKFAST		LUNCH		DINNER		BEDTIME	
Wednesday	BEFORE	AFTER	BEFORE	AFTER	BEFORE	AFTER	BEFORE	AFTER
BLOOD SUGAR								
BLOOD PRESSURE								
Date __/__/__	BREAKFAST		LUNCH		DINNER		BEDTIME	
Thursday	BEFORE	AFTER	BEFORE	AFTER	BEFORE	AFTER	BEFORE	AFTER
BLOOD SUGAR								
BLOOD PRESSURE								
Date __/__/__	BREAKFAST		LUNCH		DINNER		BEDTIME	
Friday	BEFORE	AFTER	BEFORE	AFTER	BEFORE	AFTER	BEFORE	AFTER
BLOOD SUGAR								
BLOOD PRESSURE								
Date __/__/__	BREAKFAST		LUNCH		DINNER		BEDTIME	
Saturday	BEFORE	AFTER	BEFORE	AFTER	BEFORE	AFTER	BEFORE	AFTER
BLOOD SUGAR								
BLOOD PRESSURE								
Date __/__/__	BREAKFAST		LUNCH		DINNER		BEDTIME	
Sunday	BEFORE	AFTER	BEFORE	AFTER	BEFORE	AFTER	BEFORE	AFTER
BLOOD SUGAR								
BLOOD PRESSURE								

NOTES: _____

_____

_____

_____

Month: _____ **Week Commencing:** _____

Date __/__/__	BREAKFAST		LUNCH		DINNER		BEDTIME	
Monday	BEFORE	AFTER	BEFORE	AFTER	BEFORE	AFTER	BEFORE	AFTER
BLOOD SUGAR								
BLOOD PRESSURE								

Date __/__/__	BREAKFAST		LUNCH		DINNER		BEDTIME	
Tuesday	BEFORE	AFTER	BEFORE	AFTER	BEFORE	AFTER	BEFORE	AFTER
BLOOD SUGAR								
BLOOD PRESSURE								

Date __/__/__	BREAKFAST		LUNCH		DINNER		BEDTIME	
Wednesday	BEFORE	AFTER	BEFORE	AFTER	BEFORE	AFTER	BEFORE	AFTER
BLOOD SUGAR								
BLOOD PRESSURE								

Date __/__/__	BREAKFAST		LUNCH		DINNER		BEDTIME	
Thursday	BEFORE	AFTER	BEFORE	AFTER	BEFORE	AFTER	BEFORE	AFTER
BLOOD SUGAR								
BLOOD PRESSURE								

Date __/__/__	BREAKFAST		LUNCH		DINNER		BEDTIME	
Friday	BEFORE	AFTER	BEFORE	AFTER	BEFORE	AFTER	BEFORE	AFTER
BLOOD SUGAR								
BLOOD PRESSURE								

Date __/__/__	BREAKFAST		LUNCH		DINNER		BEDTIME	
Saturday	BEFORE	AFTER	BEFORE	AFTER	BEFORE	AFTER	BEFORE	AFTER
BLOOD SUGAR								
BLOOD PRESSURE								

Date __/__/__	BREAKFAST		LUNCH		DINNER		BEDTIME	
Sunday	BEFORE	AFTER	BEFORE	AFTER	BEFORE	AFTER	BEFORE	AFTER
BLOOD SUGAR								
BLOOD PRESSURE								

NOTES: _____
_____
_____
_____

Month: _____ **Week Commencing:** _____

Date __/__/__	BREAKFAST		LUNCH		DINNER		BEDTIME	
Monday	BEFORE	AFTER	BEFORE	AFTER	BEFORE	AFTER	BEFORE	AFTER
BLOOD SUGAR								
BLOOD PRESSURE								
Date __/__/__	BREAKFAST		LUNCH		DINNER		BEDTIME	
Tuesday	BEFORE	AFTER	BEFORE	AFTER	BEFORE	AFTER	BEFORE	AFTER
BLOOD SUGAR								
BLOOD PRESSURE								
Date __/__/__	BREAKFAST		LUNCH		DINNER		BEDTIME	
Wednesday	BEFORE	AFTER	BEFORE	AFTER	BEFORE	AFTER	BEFORE	AFTER
BLOOD SUGAR								
BLOOD PRESSURE								
Date __/__/__	BREAKFAST		LUNCH		DINNER		BEDTIME	
Thursday	BEFORE	AFTER	BEFORE	AFTER	BEFORE	AFTER	BEFORE	AFTER
BLOOD SUGAR								
BLOOD PRESSURE								
Date __/__/__	BREAKFAST		LUNCH		DINNER		BEDTIME	
Friday	BEFORE	AFTER	BEFORE	AFTER	BEFORE	AFTER	BEFORE	AFTER
BLOOD SUGAR								
BLOOD PRESSURE								
Date __/__/__	BREAKFAST		LUNCH		DINNER		BEDTIME	
Saturday	BEFORE	AFTER	BEFORE	AFTER	BEFORE	AFTER	BEFORE	AFTER
BLOOD SUGAR								
BLOOD PRESSURE								
Date __/__/__	BREAKFAST		LUNCH		DINNER		BEDTIME	
Sunday	BEFORE	AFTER	BEFORE	AFTER	BEFORE	AFTER	BEFORE	AFTER
BLOOD SUGAR								
BLOOD PRESSURE								

NOTES: _____
_____
_____
_____

Month: _____ **Week Commencing:** _____

Date __/__/__	BREAKFAST		LUNCH		DINNER		BEDTIME	
Monday	BEFORE	AFTER	BEFORE	AFTER	BEFORE	AFTER	BEFORE	AFTER
BLOOD SUGAR								
BLOOD PRESSURE								
Date __/__/__	BREAKFAST		LUNCH		DINNER		BEDTIME	
Tuesday	BEFORE	AFTER	BEFORE	AFTER	BEFORE	AFTER	BEFORE	AFTER
BLOOD SUGAR								
BLOOD PRESSURE								
Date __/__/__	BREAKFAST		LUNCH		DINNER		BEDTIME	
Wednesday	BEFORE	AFTER	BEFORE	AFTER	BEFORE	AFTER	BEFORE	AFTER
BLOOD SUGAR								
BLOOD PRESSURE								
Date __/__/__	BREAKFAST		LUNCH		DINNER		BEDTIME	
Thursday	BEFORE	AFTER	BEFORE	AFTER	BEFORE	AFTER	BEFORE	AFTER
BLOOD SUGAR								
BLOOD PRESSURE								
Date __/__/__	BREAKFAST		LUNCH		DINNER		BEDTIME	
Friday	BEFORE	AFTER	BEFORE	AFTER	BEFORE	AFTER	BEFORE	AFTER
BLOOD SUGAR								
BLOOD PRESSURE								
Date __/__/__	BREAKFAST		LUNCH		DINNER		BEDTIME	
Saturday	BEFORE	AFTER	BEFORE	AFTER	BEFORE	AFTER	BEFORE	AFTER
BLOOD SUGAR								
BLOOD PRESSURE								
Date __/__/__	BREAKFAST		LUNCH		DINNER		BEDTIME	
Sunday	BEFORE	AFTER	BEFORE	AFTER	BEFORE	AFTER	BEFORE	AFTER
BLOOD SUGAR								
BLOOD PRESSURE								

NOTES: _____
_____
_____
_____

Month: _____ **Week Commencing:** _____

Date __/__/__	BREAKFAST		LUNCH		DINNER		BEDTIME	
Monday	BEFORE	AFTER	BEFORE	AFTER	BEFORE	AFTER	BEFORE	AFTER
BLOOD SUGAR								
BLOOD PRESSURE								
Date __/__/__	BREAKFAST		LUNCH		DINNER		BEDTIME	
Tuesday	BEFORE	AFTER	BEFORE	AFTER	BEFORE	AFTER	BEFORE	AFTER
BLOOD SUGAR								
BLOOD PRESSURE								
Date __/__/__	BREAKFAST		LUNCH		DINNER		BEDTIME	
Wednesday	BEFORE	AFTER	BEFORE	AFTER	BEFORE	AFTER	BEFORE	AFTER
BLOOD SUGAR								
BLOOD PRESSURE								
Date __/__/__	BREAKFAST		LUNCH		DINNER		BEDTIME	
Thursday	BEFORE	AFTER	BEFORE	AFTER	BEFORE	AFTER	BEFORE	AFTER
BLOOD SUGAR								
BLOOD PRESSURE								
Date __/__/__	BREAKFAST		LUNCH		DINNER		BEDTIME	
Friday	BEFORE	AFTER	BEFORE	AFTER	BEFORE	AFTER	BEFORE	AFTER
BLOOD SUGAR								
BLOOD PRESSURE								
Date __/__/__	BREAKFAST		LUNCH		DINNER		BEDTIME	
Saturday	BEFORE	AFTER	BEFORE	AFTER	BEFORE	AFTER	BEFORE	AFTER
BLOOD SUGAR								
BLOOD PRESSURE								
Date __/__/__	BREAKFAST		LUNCH		DINNER		BEDTIME	
Sunday	BEFORE	AFTER	BEFORE	AFTER	BEFORE	AFTER	BEFORE	AFTER
BLOOD SUGAR								
BLOOD PRESSURE								

NOTES: _____
_____
_____
_____

Month: _____ **Week Commencing:** _____

Date __/__/__	BREAKFAST		LUNCH		DINNER		BEDTIME	
Monday	BEFORE	AFTER	BEFORE	AFTER	BEFORE	AFTER	BEFORE	AFTER
BLOOD SUGAR								
BLOOD PRESSURE								
Date __/__/__	BREAKFAST		LUNCH		DINNER		BEDTIME	
Tuesday	BEFORE	AFTER	BEFORE	AFTER	BEFORE	AFTER	BEFORE	AFTER
BLOOD SUGAR								
BLOOD PRESSURE								
Date __/__/__	BREAKFAST		LUNCH		DINNER		BEDTIME	
Wednesday	BEFORE	AFTER	BEFORE	AFTER	BEFORE	AFTER	BEFORE	AFTER
BLOOD SUGAR								
BLOOD PRESSURE								
Date __/__/__	BREAKFAST		LUNCH		DINNER		BEDTIME	
Thursday	BEFORE	AFTER	BEFORE	AFTER	BEFORE	AFTER	BEFORE	AFTER
BLOOD SUGAR								
BLOOD PRESSURE								
Date __/__/__	BREAKFAST		LUNCH		DINNER		BEDTIME	
Friday	BEFORE	AFTER	BEFORE	AFTER	BEFORE	AFTER	BEFORE	AFTER
BLOOD SUGAR								
BLOOD PRESSURE								
Date __/__/__	BREAKFAST		LUNCH		DINNER		BEDTIME	
Saturday	BEFORE	AFTER	BEFORE	AFTER	BEFORE	AFTER	BEFORE	AFTER
BLOOD SUGAR								
BLOOD PRESSURE								
Date __/__/__	BREAKFAST		LUNCH		DINNER		BEDTIME	
Sunday	BEFORE	AFTER	BEFORE	AFTER	BEFORE	AFTER	BEFORE	AFTER
BLOOD SUGAR								
BLOOD PRESSURE								

NOTES: _____
_____
_____
_____

Month: _____ **Week Commencing:** _____

Date __/__/__	BREAKFAST		LUNCH		DINNER		BEDTIME	
Monday	BEFORE	AFTER	BEFORE	AFTER	BEFORE	AFTER	BEFORE	AFTER
BLOOD SUGAR								
BLOOD PRESSURE								
Date __/__/__	BREAKFAST		LUNCH		DINNER		BEDTIME	
Tuesday	BEFORE	AFTER	BEFORE	AFTER	BEFORE	AFTER	BEFORE	AFTER
BLOOD SUGAR								
BLOOD PRESSURE								
Date __/__/__	BREAKFAST		LUNCH		DINNER		BEDTIME	
Wednesday	BEFORE	AFTER	BEFORE	AFTER	BEFORE	AFTER	BEFORE	AFTER
BLOOD SUGAR								
BLOOD PRESSURE								
Date __/__/__	BREAKFAST		LUNCH		DINNER		BEDTIME	
Thursday	BEFORE	AFTER	BEFORE	AFTER	BEFORE	AFTER	BEFORE	AFTER
BLOOD SUGAR								
BLOOD PRESSURE								
Date __/__/__	BREAKFAST		LUNCH		DINNER		BEDTIME	
Friday	BEFORE	AFTER	BEFORE	AFTER	BEFORE	AFTER	BEFORE	AFTER
BLOOD SUGAR								
BLOOD PRESSURE								
Date __/__/__	BREAKFAST		LUNCH		DINNER		BEDTIME	
Saturday	BEFORE	AFTER	BEFORE	AFTER	BEFORE	AFTER	BEFORE	AFTER
BLOOD SUGAR								
BLOOD PRESSURE								
Date __/__/__	BREAKFAST		LUNCH		DINNER		BEDTIME	
Sunday	BEFORE	AFTER	BEFORE	AFTER	BEFORE	AFTER	BEFORE	AFTER
BLOOD SUGAR								
BLOOD PRESSURE								

NOTES: _____
_____
_____
_____

Month: _____ **Week Commencing:** _____

Date __/__/__	BREAKFAST		LUNCH		DINNER		BEDTIME	
Monday	BEFORE	AFTER	BEFORE	AFTER	BEFORE	AFTER	BEFORE	AFTER
BLOOD SUGAR								
BLOOD PRESSURE								
Date __/__/__	BREAKFAST		LUNCH		DINNER		BEDTIME	
Tuesday	BEFORE	AFTER	BEFORE	AFTER	BEFORE	AFTER	BEFORE	AFTER
BLOOD SUGAR								
BLOOD PRESSURE								
Date __/__/__	BREAKFAST		LUNCH		DINNER		BEDTIME	
Wednesday	BEFORE	AFTER	BEFORE	AFTER	BEFORE	AFTER	BEFORE	AFTER
BLOOD SUGAR								
BLOOD PRESSURE								
Date __/__/__	BREAKFAST		LUNCH		DINNER		BEDTIME	
Thursday	BEFORE	AFTER	BEFORE	AFTER	BEFORE	AFTER	BEFORE	AFTER
BLOOD SUGAR								
BLOOD PRESSURE								
Date __/__/__	BREAKFAST		LUNCH		DINNER		BEDTIME	
Friday	BEFORE	AFTER	BEFORE	AFTER	BEFORE	AFTER	BEFORE	AFTER
BLOOD SUGAR								
BLOOD PRESSURE								
Date __/__/__	BREAKFAST		LUNCH		DINNER		BEDTIME	
Saturday	BEFORE	AFTER	BEFORE	AFTER	BEFORE	AFTER	BEFORE	AFTER
BLOOD SUGAR								
BLOOD PRESSURE								
Date __/__/__	BREAKFAST		LUNCH		DINNER		BEDTIME	
Sunday	BEFORE	AFTER	BEFORE	AFTER	BEFORE	AFTER	BEFORE	AFTER
BLOOD SUGAR								
BLOOD PRESSURE								

NOTES: _____

_____

_____

Month: _____ **Week Commencing:** _____

Date __/__/__	BREAKFAST		LUNCH		DINNER		BEDTIME	
Monday	BEFORE	AFTER	BEFORE	AFTER	BEFORE	AFTER	BEFORE	AFTER
BLOOD SUGAR								
BLOOD PRESSURE								
Date __/__/__	BREAKFAST		LUNCH		DINNER		BEDTIME	
Tuesday	BEFORE	AFTER	BEFORE	AFTER	BEFORE	AFTER	BEFORE	AFTER
BLOOD SUGAR								
BLOOD PRESSURE								
Date __/__/__	BREAKFAST		LUNCH		DINNER		BEDTIME	
Wednesday	BEFORE	AFTER	BEFORE	AFTER	BEFORE	AFTER	BEFORE	AFTER
BLOOD SUGAR								
BLOOD PRESSURE								
Date __/__/__	BREAKFAST		LUNCH		DINNER		BEDTIME	
Thursday	BEFORE	AFTER	BEFORE	AFTER	BEFORE	AFTER	BEFORE	AFTER
BLOOD SUGAR								
BLOOD PRESSURE								
Date __/__/__	BREAKFAST		LUNCH		DINNER		BEDTIME	
Friday	BEFORE	AFTER	BEFORE	AFTER	BEFORE	AFTER	BEFORE	AFTER
BLOOD SUGAR								
BLOOD PRESSURE								
Date __/__/__	BREAKFAST		LUNCH		DINNER		BEDTIME	
Saturday	BEFORE	AFTER	BEFORE	AFTER	BEFORE	AFTER	BEFORE	AFTER
BLOOD SUGAR								
BLOOD PRESSURE								
Date __/__/__	BREAKFAST		LUNCH		DINNER		BEDTIME	
Sunday	BEFORE	AFTER	BEFORE	AFTER	BEFORE	AFTER	BEFORE	AFTER
BLOOD SUGAR								
BLOOD PRESSURE								

NOTES: _____
_____
_____
_____

Month: _____ **Week Commencing:** _____

Date __/__/__	BREAKFAST		LUNCH		DINNER		BEDTIME	
Monday	BEFORE	AFTER	BEFORE	AFTER	BEFORE	AFTER	BEFORE	AFTER
BLOOD SUGAR								
BLOOD PRESSURE								
Date __/__/__	BREAKFAST		LUNCH		DINNER		BEDTIME	
Tuesday	BEFORE	AFTER	BEFORE	AFTER	BEFORE	AFTER	BEFORE	AFTER
BLOOD SUGAR								
BLOOD PRESSURE								
Date __/__/__	BREAKFAST		LUNCH		DINNER		BEDTIME	
Wednesday	BEFORE	AFTER	BEFORE	AFTER	BEFORE	AFTER	BEFORE	AFTER
BLOOD SUGAR								
BLOOD PRESSURE								
Date __/__/__	BREAKFAST		LUNCH		DINNER		BEDTIME	
Thursday	BEFORE	AFTER	BEFORE	AFTER	BEFORE	AFTER	BEFORE	AFTER
BLOOD SUGAR								
BLOOD PRESSURE								
Date __/__/__	BREAKFAST		LUNCH		DINNER		BEDTIME	
Friday	BEFORE	AFTER	BEFORE	AFTER	BEFORE	AFTER	BEFORE	AFTER
BLOOD SUGAR								
BLOOD PRESSURE								
Date __/__/__	BREAKFAST		LUNCH		DINNER		BEDTIME	
Saturday	BEFORE	AFTER	BEFORE	AFTER	BEFORE	AFTER	BEFORE	AFTER
BLOOD SUGAR								
BLOOD PRESSURE								
Date __/__/__	BREAKFAST		LUNCH		DINNER		BEDTIME	
Sunday	BEFORE	AFTER	BEFORE	AFTER	BEFORE	AFTER	BEFORE	AFTER
BLOOD SUGAR								
BLOOD PRESSURE								

NOTES: _____
_____
_____
_____

Month: _____ **Week Commencing:** _____

Date __/__/__	BREAKFAST		LUNCH		DINNER		BEDTIME	
Monday	BEFORE	AFTER	BEFORE	AFTER	BEFORE	AFTER	BEFORE	AFTER
BLOOD SUGAR								
BLOOD PRESSURE								
Date __/__/__	BREAKFAST		LUNCH		DINNER		BEDTIME	
Tuesday	BEFORE	AFTER	BEFORE	AFTER	BEFORE	AFTER	BEFORE	AFTER
BLOOD SUGAR								
BLOOD PRESSURE								
Date __/__/__	BREAKFAST		LUNCH		DINNER		BEDTIME	
Wednesday	BEFORE	AFTER	BEFORE	AFTER	BEFORE	AFTER	BEFORE	AFTER
BLOOD SUGAR								
BLOOD PRESSURE								
Date __/__/__	BREAKFAST		LUNCH		DINNER		BEDTIME	
Thursday	BEFORE	AFTER	BEFORE	AFTER	BEFORE	AFTER	BEFORE	AFTER
BLOOD SUGAR								
BLOOD PRESSURE								
Date __/__/__	BREAKFAST		LUNCH		DINNER		BEDTIME	
Friday	BEFORE	AFTER	BEFORE	AFTER	BEFORE	AFTER	BEFORE	AFTER
BLOOD SUGAR								
BLOOD PRESSURE								
Date __/__/__	BREAKFAST		LUNCH		DINNER		BEDTIME	
Saturday	BEFORE	AFTER	BEFORE	AFTER	BEFORE	AFTER	BEFORE	AFTER
BLOOD SUGAR								
BLOOD PRESSURE								
Date __/__/__	BREAKFAST		LUNCH		DINNER		BEDTIME	
Sunday	BEFORE	AFTER	BEFORE	AFTER	BEFORE	AFTER	BEFORE	AFTER
BLOOD SUGAR								
BLOOD PRESSURE								

NOTES: _____
_____
_____
_____

Month: _____ **Week Commencing:** _____

Date __/__/__	BREAKFAST		LUNCH		DINNER		BEDTIME	
Monday	BEFORE	AFTER	BEFORE	AFTER	BEFORE	AFTER	BEFORE	AFTER
BLOOD SUGAR								
BLOOD PRESSURE								
Date __/__/__	BREAKFAST		LUNCH		DINNER		BEDTIME	
Tuesday	BEFORE	AFTER	BEFORE	AFTER	BEFORE	AFTER	BEFORE	AFTER
BLOOD SUGAR								
BLOOD PRESSURE								
Date __/__/__	BREAKFAST		LUNCH		DINNER		BEDTIME	
Wednesday	BEFORE	AFTER	BEFORE	AFTER	BEFORE	AFTER	BEFORE	AFTER
BLOOD SUGAR								
BLOOD PRESSURE								
Date __/__/__	BREAKFAST		LUNCH		DINNER		BEDTIME	
Thursday	BEFORE	AFTER	BEFORE	AFTER	BEFORE	AFTER	BEFORE	AFTER
BLOOD SUGAR								
BLOOD PRESSURE								
Date __/__/__	BREAKFAST		LUNCH		DINNER		BEDTIME	
Friday	BEFORE	AFTER	BEFORE	AFTER	BEFORE	AFTER	BEFORE	AFTER
BLOOD SUGAR								
BLOOD PRESSURE								
Date __/__/__	BREAKFAST		LUNCH		DINNER		BEDTIME	
Saturday	BEFORE	AFTER	BEFORE	AFTER	BEFORE	AFTER	BEFORE	AFTER
BLOOD SUGAR								
BLOOD PRESSURE								
Date __/__/__	BREAKFAST		LUNCH		DINNER		BEDTIME	
Sunday	BEFORE	AFTER	BEFORE	AFTER	BEFORE	AFTER	BEFORE	AFTER
BLOOD SUGAR								
BLOOD PRESSURE								

NOTES: _____
_____
_____

Month: _____ **Week Commencing:** _____

Date __/__/__	BREAKFAST		LUNCH		DINNER		BEDTIME	
Monday	BEFORE	AFTER	BEFORE	AFTER	BEFORE	AFTER	BEFORE	AFTER
BLOOD SUGAR								
BLOOD PRESSURE								
Date __/__/__	BREAKFAST		LUNCH		DINNER		BEDTIME	
Tuesday	BEFORE	AFTER	BEFORE	AFTER	BEFORE	AFTER	BEFORE	AFTER
BLOOD SUGAR								
BLOOD PRESSURE								
Date __/__/__	BREAKFAST		LUNCH		DINNER		BEDTIME	
Wednesday	BEFORE	AFTER	BEFORE	AFTER	BEFORE	AFTER	BEFORE	AFTER
BLOOD SUGAR								
BLOOD PRESSURE								
Date __/__/__	BREAKFAST		LUNCH		DINNER		BEDTIME	
Thursday	BEFORE	AFTER	BEFORE	AFTER	BEFORE	AFTER	BEFORE	AFTER
BLOOD SUGAR								
BLOOD PRESSURE								
Date __/__/__	BREAKFAST		LUNCH		DINNER		BEDTIME	
Friday	BEFORE	AFTER	BEFORE	AFTER	BEFORE	AFTER	BEFORE	AFTER
BLOOD SUGAR								
BLOOD PRESSURE								
Date __/__/__	BREAKFAST		LUNCH		DINNER		BEDTIME	
Saturday	BEFORE	AFTER	BEFORE	AFTER	BEFORE	AFTER	BEFORE	AFTER
BLOOD SUGAR								
BLOOD PRESSURE								
Date __/__/__	BREAKFAST		LUNCH		DINNER		BEDTIME	
Sunday	BEFORE	AFTER	BEFORE	AFTER	BEFORE	AFTER	BEFORE	AFTER
BLOOD SUGAR								
BLOOD PRESSURE								

NOTES: _____
_____
_____
_____

Month: _____ **Week Commencing:** _____

Date ___/___/___	BREAKFAST		LUNCH		DINNER		BEDTIME	
Monday	BEFORE	AFTER	BEFORE	AFTER	BEFORE	AFTER	BEFORE	AFTER
BLOOD SUGAR								
BLOOD PRESSURE								

Date ___/___/___	BREAKFAST		LUNCH		DINNER		BEDTIME	
Tuesday	BEFORE	AFTER	BEFORE	AFTER	BEFORE	AFTER	BEFORE	AFTER
BLOOD SUGAR								
BLOOD PRESSURE								

Date ___/___/___	BREAKFAST		LUNCH		DINNER		BEDTIME	
Wednesday	BEFORE	AFTER	BEFORE	AFTER	BEFORE	AFTER	BEFORE	AFTER
BLOOD SUGAR								
BLOOD PRESSURE								

Date ___/___/___	BREAKFAST		LUNCH		DINNER		BEDTIME	
Thursday	BEFORE	AFTER	BEFORE	AFTER	BEFORE	AFTER	BEFORE	AFTER
BLOOD SUGAR								
BLOOD PRESSURE								

Date ___/___/___	BREAKFAST		LUNCH		DINNER		BEDTIME	
Friday	BEFORE	AFTER	BEFORE	AFTER	BEFORE	AFTER	BEFORE	AFTER
BLOOD SUGAR								
BLOOD PRESSURE								

Date ___/___/___	BREAKFAST		LUNCH		DINNER		BEDTIME	
Saturday	BEFORE	AFTER	BEFORE	AFTER	BEFORE	AFTER	BEFORE	AFTER
BLOOD SUGAR								
BLOOD PRESSURE								

Date ___/___/___	BREAKFAST		LUNCH		DINNER		BEDTIME	
Sunday	BEFORE	AFTER	BEFORE	AFTER	BEFORE	AFTER	BEFORE	AFTER
BLOOD SUGAR								
BLOOD PRESSURE								

NOTES: _____
_____
_____
_____

Month: _____ **Week Commencing:** _____

Date __/__/__ Monday	BREAKFAST		LUNCH		DINNER		BEDTIME	
	BEFORE	AFTER	BEFORE	AFTER	BEFORE	AFTER	BEFORE	AFTER
BLOOD SUGAR								
BLOOD PRESSURE								

Date __/__/__ Tuesday	BREAKFAST		LUNCH		DINNER		BEDTIME	
	BEFORE	AFTER	BEFORE	AFTER	BEFORE	AFTER	BEFORE	AFTER
BLOOD SUGAR								
BLOOD PRESSURE								

Date __/__/__ Wednesday	BREAKFAST		LUNCH		DINNER		BEDTIME	
	BEFORE	AFTER	BEFORE	AFTER	BEFORE	AFTER	BEFORE	AFTER
BLOOD SUGAR								
BLOOD PRESSURE								

Date __/__/__ Thursday	BREAKFAST		LUNCH		DINNER		BEDTIME	
	BEFORE	AFTER	BEFORE	AFTER	BEFORE	AFTER	BEFORE	AFTER
BLOOD SUGAR								
BLOOD PRESSURE								

Date __/__/__ Friday	BREAKFAST		LUNCH		DINNER		BEDTIME	
	BEFORE	AFTER	BEFORE	AFTER	BEFORE	AFTER	BEFORE	AFTER
BLOOD SUGAR								
BLOOD PRESSURE								

Date __/__/__ Saturday	BREAKFAST		LUNCH		DINNER		BEDTIME	
	BEFORE	AFTER	BEFORE	AFTER	BEFORE	AFTER	BEFORE	AFTER
BLOOD SUGAR								
BLOOD PRESSURE								

Date __/__/__ Sunday	BREAKFAST		LUNCH		DINNER		BEDTIME	
	BEFORE	AFTER	BEFORE	AFTER	BEFORE	AFTER	BEFORE	AFTER
BLOOD SUGAR								
BLOOD PRESSURE								

NOTES: _____
_____
_____
_____

Month: _____ **Week Commencing:** _____

Date __/__/__	BREAKFAST		LUNCH		DINNER		BEDTIME	
Monday	BEFORE	AFTER	BEFORE	AFTER	BEFORE	AFTER	BEFORE	AFTER
BLOOD SUGAR								
BLOOD PRESSURE								
Date __/__/__	BREAKFAST		LUNCH		DINNER		BEDTIME	
Tuesday	BEFORE	AFTER	BEFORE	AFTER	BEFORE	AFTER	BEFORE	AFTER
BLOOD SUGAR								
BLOOD PRESSURE								
Date __/__/__	BREAKFAST		LUNCH		DINNER		BEDTIME	
Wednesday	BEFORE	AFTER	BEFORE	AFTER	BEFORE	AFTER	BEFORE	AFTER
BLOOD SUGAR								
BLOOD PRESSURE								
Date __/__/__	BREAKFAST		LUNCH		DINNER		BEDTIME	
Thursday	BEFORE	AFTER	BEFORE	AFTER	BEFORE	AFTER	BEFORE	AFTER
BLOOD SUGAR								
BLOOD PRESSURE								
Date __/__/__	BREAKFAST		LUNCH		DINNER		BEDTIME	
Friday	BEFORE	AFTER	BEFORE	AFTER	BEFORE	AFTER	BEFORE	AFTER
BLOOD SUGAR								
BLOOD PRESSURE								
Date __/__/__	BREAKFAST		LUNCH		DINNER		BEDTIME	
Saturday	BEFORE	AFTER	BEFORE	AFTER	BEFORE	AFTER	BEFORE	AFTER
BLOOD SUGAR								
BLOOD PRESSURE								
Date __/__/__	BREAKFAST		LUNCH		DINNER		BEDTIME	
Sunday	BEFORE	AFTER	BEFORE	AFTER	BEFORE	AFTER	BEFORE	AFTER
BLOOD SUGAR								
BLOOD PRESSURE								

NOTES: _____
_____
_____
_____

Month: _____ **Week Commencing:** _____

Date __/__/__ Monday	BREAKFAST		LUNCH		DINNER		BEDTIME	
	BEFORE	AFTER	BEFORE	AFTER	BEFORE	AFTER	BEFORE	AFTER
BLOOD SUGAR								
BLOOD PRESSURE								

Date __/__/__ Tuesday	BREAKFAST		LUNCH		DINNER		BEDTIME	
	BEFORE	AFTER	BEFORE	AFTER	BEFORE	AFTER	BEFORE	AFTER
BLOOD SUGAR								
BLOOD PRESSURE								

Date __/__/__ Wednesday	BREAKFAST		LUNCH		DINNER		BEDTIME	
	BEFORE	AFTER	BEFORE	AFTER	BEFORE	AFTER	BEFORE	AFTER
BLOOD SUGAR								
BLOOD PRESSURE								

Date __/__/__ Thursday	BREAKFAST		LUNCH		DINNER		BEDTIME	
	BEFORE	AFTER	BEFORE	AFTER	BEFORE	AFTER	BEFORE	AFTER
BLOOD SUGAR								
BLOOD PRESSURE								

Date __/__/__ Friday	BREAKFAST		LUNCH		DINNER		BEDTIME	
	BEFORE	AFTER	BEFORE	AFTER	BEFORE	AFTER	BEFORE	AFTER
BLOOD SUGAR								
BLOOD PRESSURE								

Date __/__/__ Saturday	BREAKFAST		LUNCH		DINNER		BEDTIME	
	BEFORE	AFTER	BEFORE	AFTER	BEFORE	AFTER	BEFORE	AFTER
BLOOD SUGAR								
BLOOD PRESSURE								

Date __/__/__ Sunday	BREAKFAST		LUNCH		DINNER		BEDTIME	
	BEFORE	AFTER	BEFORE	AFTER	BEFORE	AFTER	BEFORE	AFTER
BLOOD SUGAR								
BLOOD PRESSURE								

NOTES: _____
_____
_____
_____

Month: _____ **Week Commencing:** _____

Date __/__/__	BREAKFAST		LUNCH		DINNER		BEDTIME	
Monday	BEFORE	AFTER	BEFORE	AFTER	BEFORE	AFTER	BEFORE	AFTER
BLOOD SUGAR								
BLOOD PRESSURE								
Date __/__/__	BREAKFAST		LUNCH		DINNER		BEDTIME	
Tuesday	BEFORE	AFTER	BEFORE	AFTER	BEFORE	AFTER	BEFORE	AFTER
BLOOD SUGAR								
BLOOD PRESSURE								
Date __/__/__	BREAKFAST		LUNCH		DINNER		BEDTIME	
Wednesday	BEFORE	AFTER	BEFORE	AFTER	BEFORE	AFTER	BEFORE	AFTER
BLOOD SUGAR								
BLOOD PRESSURE								
Date __/__/__	BREAKFAST		LUNCH		DINNER		BEDTIME	
Thursday	BEFORE	AFTER	BEFORE	AFTER	BEFORE	AFTER	BEFORE	AFTER
BLOOD SUGAR								
BLOOD PRESSURE								
Date __/__/__	BREAKFAST		LUNCH		DINNER		BEDTIME	
Friday	BEFORE	AFTER	BEFORE	AFTER	BEFORE	AFTER	BEFORE	AFTER
BLOOD SUGAR								
BLOOD PRESSURE								
Date __/__/__	BREAKFAST		LUNCH		DINNER		BEDTIME	
Saturday	BEFORE	AFTER	BEFORE	AFTER	BEFORE	AFTER	BEFORE	AFTER
BLOOD SUGAR								
BLOOD PRESSURE								
Date __/__/__	BREAKFAST		LUNCH		DINNER		BEDTIME	
Sunday	BEFORE	AFTER	BEFORE	AFTER	BEFORE	AFTER	BEFORE	AFTER
BLOOD SUGAR								
BLOOD PRESSURE								

NOTES: _____
_____
_____
_____

Month: _____ **Week Commencing:** _____

Date __/__/__ Monday	BREAKFAST		LUNCH		DINNER		BEDTIME	
	BEFORE	AFTER	BEFORE	AFTER	BEFORE	AFTER	BEFORE	AFTER
BLOOD SUGAR								
BLOOD PRESSURE								

Date __/__/__ Tuesday	BREAKFAST		LUNCH		DINNER		BEDTIME	
	BEFORE	AFTER	BEFORE	AFTER	BEFORE	AFTER	BEFORE	AFTER
BLOOD SUGAR								
BLOOD PRESSURE								

Date __/__/__ Wednesday	BREAKFAST		LUNCH		DINNER		BEDTIME	
	BEFORE	AFTER	BEFORE	AFTER	BEFORE	AFTER	BEFORE	AFTER
BLOOD SUGAR								
BLOOD PRESSURE								

Date __/__/__ Thursday	BREAKFAST		LUNCH		DINNER		BEDTIME	
	BEFORE	AFTER	BEFORE	AFTER	BEFORE	AFTER	BEFORE	AFTER
BLOOD SUGAR								
BLOOD PRESSURE								

Date __/__/__ Friday	BREAKFAST		LUNCH		DINNER		BEDTIME	
	BEFORE	AFTER	BEFORE	AFTER	BEFORE	AFTER	BEFORE	AFTER
BLOOD SUGAR								
BLOOD PRESSURE								

Date __/__/__ Saturday	BREAKFAST		LUNCH		DINNER		BEDTIME	
	BEFORE	AFTER	BEFORE	AFTER	BEFORE	AFTER	BEFORE	AFTER
BLOOD SUGAR								
BLOOD PRESSURE								

Date __/__/__ Sunday	BREAKFAST		LUNCH		DINNER		BEDTIME	
	BEFORE	AFTER	BEFORE	AFTER	BEFORE	AFTER	BEFORE	AFTER
BLOOD SUGAR								
BLOOD PRESSURE								

NOTES: _____
_____
_____

Month: _____ **Week Commencing:** _____

Date ___/___/___	BREAKFAST		LUNCH		DINNER		BEDTIME	
Monday	BEFORE	AFTER	BEFORE	AFTER	BEFORE	AFTER	BEFORE	AFTER
BLOOD SUGAR								
BLOOD PRESSURE								
Date ___/___/___	BREAKFAST		LUNCH		DINNER		BEDTIME	
Tuesday	BEFORE	AFTER	BEFORE	AFTER	BEFORE	AFTER	BEFORE	AFTER
BLOOD SUGAR								
BLOOD PRESSURE								
Date ___/___/___	BREAKFAST		LUNCH		DINNER		BEDTIME	
Wednesday	BEFORE	AFTER	BEFORE	AFTER	BEFORE	AFTER	BEFORE	AFTER
BLOOD SUGAR								
BLOOD PRESSURE								
Date ___/___/___	BREAKFAST		LUNCH		DINNER		BEDTIME	
Thursday	BEFORE	AFTER	BEFORE	AFTER	BEFORE	AFTER	BEFORE	AFTER
BLOOD SUGAR								
BLOOD PRESSURE								
Date ___/___/___	BREAKFAST		LUNCH		DINNER		BEDTIME	
Friday	BEFORE	AFTER	BEFORE	AFTER	BEFORE	AFTER	BEFORE	AFTER
BLOOD SUGAR								
BLOOD PRESSURE								
Date ___/___/___	BREAKFAST		LUNCH		DINNER		BEDTIME	
Saturday	BEFORE	AFTER	BEFORE	AFTER	BEFORE	AFTER	BEFORE	AFTER
BLOOD SUGAR								
BLOOD PRESSURE								
Date ___/___/___	BREAKFAST		LUNCH		DINNER		BEDTIME	
Sunday	BEFORE	AFTER	BEFORE	AFTER	BEFORE	AFTER	BEFORE	AFTER
BLOOD SUGAR								
BLOOD PRESSURE								

NOTES: _____
_____
_____
_____

Month: _____ **Week Commencing:** _____

Date __/__/__	BREAKFAST		LUNCH		DINNER		BEDTIME	
Monday	BEFORE	AFTER	BEFORE	AFTER	BEFORE	AFTER	BEFORE	AFTER
BLOOD SUGAR								
BLOOD PRESSURE								
Date __/__/__	BREAKFAST		LUNCH		DINNER		BEDTIME	
Tuesday	BEFORE	AFTER	BEFORE	AFTER	BEFORE	AFTER	BEFORE	AFTER
BLOOD SUGAR								
BLOOD PRESSURE								
Date __/__/__	BREAKFAST		LUNCH		DINNER		BEDTIME	
Wednesday	BEFORE	AFTER	BEFORE	AFTER	BEFORE	AFTER	BEFORE	AFTER
BLOOD SUGAR								
BLOOD PRESSURE								
Date __/__/__	BREAKFAST		LUNCH		DINNER		BEDTIME	
Thursday	BEFORE	AFTER	BEFORE	AFTER	BEFORE	AFTER	BEFORE	AFTER
BLOOD SUGAR								
BLOOD PRESSURE								
Date __/__/__	BREAKFAST		LUNCH		DINNER		BEDTIME	
Friday	BEFORE	AFTER	BEFORE	AFTER	BEFORE	AFTER	BEFORE	AFTER
BLOOD SUGAR								
BLOOD PRESSURE								
Date __/__/__	BREAKFAST		LUNCH		DINNER		BEDTIME	
Saturday	BEFORE	AFTER	BEFORE	AFTER	BEFORE	AFTER	BEFORE	AFTER
BLOOD SUGAR								
BLOOD PRESSURE								
Date __/__/__	BREAKFAST		LUNCH		DINNER		BEDTIME	
Sunday	BEFORE	AFTER	BEFORE	AFTER	BEFORE	AFTER	BEFORE	AFTER
BLOOD SUGAR								
BLOOD PRESSURE								

NOTES: _____
_____
_____
_____

Month: _____ **Week Commencing:** _____

Date __/__/__	BREAKFAST		LUNCH		DINNER		BEDTIME	
Monday	BEFORE	AFTER	BEFORE	AFTER	BEFORE	AFTER	BEFORE	AFTER
BLOOD SUGAR								
BLOOD PRESSURE								
Date __/__/__	BREAKFAST		LUNCH		DINNER		BEDTIME	
Tuesday	BEFORE	AFTER	BEFORE	AFTER	BEFORE	AFTER	BEFORE	AFTER
BLOOD SUGAR								
BLOOD PRESSURE								
Date __/__/__	BREAKFAST		LUNCH		DINNER		BEDTIME	
Wednesday	BEFORE	AFTER	BEFORE	AFTER	BEFORE	AFTER	BEFORE	AFTER
BLOOD SUGAR								
BLOOD PRESSURE								
Date __/__/__	BREAKFAST		LUNCH		DINNER		BEDTIME	
Thursday	BEFORE	AFTER	BEFORE	AFTER	BEFORE	AFTER	BEFORE	AFTER
BLOOD SUGAR								
BLOOD PRESSURE								
Date __/__/__	BREAKFAST		LUNCH		DINNER		BEDTIME	
Friday	BEFORE	AFTER	BEFORE	AFTER	BEFORE	AFTER	BEFORE	AFTER
BLOOD SUGAR								
BLOOD PRESSURE								
Date __/__/__	BREAKFAST		LUNCH		DINNER		BEDTIME	
Saturday	BEFORE	AFTER	BEFORE	AFTER	BEFORE	AFTER	BEFORE	AFTER
BLOOD SUGAR								
BLOOD PRESSURE								
Date __/__/__	BREAKFAST		LUNCH		DINNER		BEDTIME	
Sunday	BEFORE	AFTER	BEFORE	AFTER	BEFORE	AFTER	BEFORE	AFTER
BLOOD SUGAR								
BLOOD PRESSURE								

NOTES: _____

_____

_____

_____

Month: _____ **Week Commencing:** _____

Date __/__/__	BREAKFAST		LUNCH		DINNER		BEDTIME	
Monday	BEFORE	AFTER	BEFORE	AFTER	BEFORE	AFTER	BEFORE	AFTER
BLOOD SUGAR								
BLOOD PRESSURE								
Date __/__/__	BREAKFAST		LUNCH		DINNER		BEDTIME	
Tuesday	BEFORE	AFTER	BEFORE	AFTER	BEFORE	AFTER	BEFORE	AFTER
BLOOD SUGAR								
BLOOD PRESSURE								
Date __/__/__	BREAKFAST		LUNCH		DINNER		BEDTIME	
Wednesday	BEFORE	AFTER	BEFORE	AFTER	BEFORE	AFTER	BEFORE	AFTER
BLOOD SUGAR								
BLOOD PRESSURE								
Date __/__/__	BREAKFAST		LUNCH		DINNER		BEDTIME	
Thursday	BEFORE	AFTER	BEFORE	AFTER	BEFORE	AFTER	BEFORE	AFTER
BLOOD SUGAR								
BLOOD PRESSURE								
Date __/__/__	BREAKFAST		LUNCH		DINNER		BEDTIME	
Friday	BEFORE	AFTER	BEFORE	AFTER	BEFORE	AFTER	BEFORE	AFTER
BLOOD SUGAR								
BLOOD PRESSURE								
Date __/__/__	BREAKFAST		LUNCH		DINNER		BEDTIME	
Saturday	BEFORE	AFTER	BEFORE	AFTER	BEFORE	AFTER	BEFORE	AFTER
BLOOD SUGAR								
BLOOD PRESSURE								
Date __/__/__	BREAKFAST		LUNCH		DINNER		BEDTIME	
Sunday	BEFORE	AFTER	BEFORE	AFTER	BEFORE	AFTER	BEFORE	AFTER
BLOOD SUGAR								
BLOOD PRESSURE								

NOTES: _____
_____
_____
_____

Month: _____ Week Commencing: _____

Date __/__/__	BREAKFAST		LUNCH		DINNER		BEDTIME	
Monday	BEFORE	AFTER	BEFORE	AFTER	BEFORE	AFTER	BEFORE	AFTER
BLOOD SUGAR								
BLOOD PRESSURE								
Date __/__/__	BREAKFAST		LUNCH		DINNER		BEDTIME	
Tuesday	BEFORE	AFTER	BEFORE	AFTER	BEFORE	AFTER	BEFORE	AFTER
BLOOD SUGAR								
BLOOD PRESSURE								
Date __/__/__	BREAKFAST		LUNCH		DINNER		BEDTIME	
Wednesday	BEFORE	AFTER	BEFORE	AFTER	BEFORE	AFTER	BEFORE	AFTER
BLOOD SUGAR								
BLOOD PRESSURE								
Date __/__/__	BREAKFAST		LUNCH		DINNER		BEDTIME	
Thursday	BEFORE	AFTER	BEFORE	AFTER	BEFORE	AFTER	BEFORE	AFTER
BLOOD SUGAR								
BLOOD PRESSURE								
Date __/__/__	BREAKFAST		LUNCH		DINNER		BEDTIME	
Friday	BEFORE	AFTER	BEFORE	AFTER	BEFORE	AFTER	BEFORE	AFTER
BLOOD SUGAR								
BLOOD PRESSURE								
Date __/__/__	BREAKFAST		LUNCH		DINNER		BEDTIME	
Saturday	BEFORE	AFTER	BEFORE	AFTER	BEFORE	AFTER	BEFORE	AFTER
BLOOD SUGAR								
BLOOD PRESSURE								
Date __/__/__	BREAKFAST		LUNCH		DINNER		BEDTIME	
Sunday	BEFORE	AFTER	BEFORE	AFTER	BEFORE	AFTER	BEFORE	AFTER
BLOOD SUGAR								
BLOOD PRESSURE								

NOTES: _____
_____
_____
_____

Month: _____ **Week Commencing:** _____

Date __/__/__ Monday	BREAKFAST		LUNCH		DINNER		BEDTIME	
	BEFORE	AFTER	BEFORE	AFTER	BEFORE	AFTER	BEFORE	AFTER
BLOOD SUGAR								
BLOOD PRESSURE								

Date __/__/__ Tuesday	BREAKFAST		LUNCH		DINNER		BEDTIME	
	BEFORE	AFTER	BEFORE	AFTER	BEFORE	AFTER	BEFORE	AFTER
BLOOD SUGAR								
BLOOD PRESSURE								

Date __/__/__ Wednesday	BREAKFAST		LUNCH		DINNER		BEDTIME	
	BEFORE	AFTER	BEFORE	AFTER	BEFORE	AFTER	BEFORE	AFTER
BLOOD SUGAR								
BLOOD PRESSURE								

Date __/__/__ Thursday	BREAKFAST		LUNCH		DINNER		BEDTIME	
	BEFORE	AFTER	BEFORE	AFTER	BEFORE	AFTER	BEFORE	AFTER
BLOOD SUGAR								
BLOOD PRESSURE								

Date __/__/__ Friday	BREAKFAST		LUNCH		DINNER		BEDTIME	
	BEFORE	AFTER	BEFORE	AFTER	BEFORE	AFTER	BEFORE	AFTER
BLOOD SUGAR								
BLOOD PRESSURE								

Date __/__/__ Saturday	BREAKFAST		LUNCH		DINNER		BEDTIME	
	BEFORE	AFTER	BEFORE	AFTER	BEFORE	AFTER	BEFORE	AFTER
BLOOD SUGAR								
BLOOD PRESSURE								

Date __/__/__ Sunday	BREAKFAST		LUNCH		DINNER		BEDTIME	
	BEFORE	AFTER	BEFORE	AFTER	BEFORE	AFTER	BEFORE	AFTER
BLOOD SUGAR								
BLOOD PRESSURE								

NOTES: _____
_____
_____
_____

Month: _____ Week Commencing: _____

Date __/__/__	BREAKFAST		LUNCH		DINNER		BEDTIME	
Monday	BEFORE	AFTER	BEFORE	AFTER	BEFORE	AFTER	BEFORE	AFTER
BLOOD SUGAR								
BLOOD PRESSURE								
Date __/__/__	BREAKFAST		LUNCH		DINNER		BEDTIME	
Tuesday	BEFORE	AFTER	BEFORE	AFTER	BEFORE	AFTER	BEFORE	AFTER
BLOOD SUGAR								
BLOOD PRESSURE								
Date __/__/__	BREAKFAST		LUNCH		DINNER		BEDTIME	
Wednesday	BEFORE	AFTER	BEFORE	AFTER	BEFORE	AFTER	BEFORE	AFTER
BLOOD SUGAR								
BLOOD PRESSURE								
Date __/__/__	BREAKFAST		LUNCH		DINNER		BEDTIME	
Thursday	BEFORE	AFTER	BEFORE	AFTER	BEFORE	AFTER	BEFORE	AFTER
BLOOD SUGAR								
BLOOD PRESSURE								
Date __/__/__	BREAKFAST		LUNCH		DINNER		BEDTIME	
Friday	BEFORE	AFTER	BEFORE	AFTER	BEFORE	AFTER	BEFORE	AFTER
BLOOD SUGAR								
BLOOD PRESSURE								
Date __/__/__	BREAKFAST		LUNCH		DINNER		BEDTIME	
Saturday	BEFORE	AFTER	BEFORE	AFTER	BEFORE	AFTER	BEFORE	AFTER
BLOOD SUGAR								
BLOOD PRESSURE								
Date __/__/__	BREAKFAST		LUNCH		DINNER		BEDTIME	
Sunday	BEFORE	AFTER	BEFORE	AFTER	BEFORE	AFTER	BEFORE	AFTER
BLOOD SUGAR								
BLOOD PRESSURE								

NOTES: _____

_____

_____

Month: _____ **Week Commencing:** _____

Date __/__/__ **Monday**	**BREAKFAST**		**LUNCH**		**DINNER**		**BEDTIME**	
	BEFORE	AFTER	BEFORE	AFTER	BEFORE	AFTER	BEFORE	AFTER
BLOOD SUGAR								
BLOOD PRESSURE								
Date __/__/__ **Tuesday**	**BREAKFAST**		**LUNCH**		**DINNER**		**BEDTIME**	
	BEFORE	AFTER	BEFORE	AFTER	BEFORE	AFTER	BEFORE	AFTER
BLOOD SUGAR								
BLOOD PRESSURE								
Date __/__/__ **Wednesday**	**BREAKFAST**		**LUNCH**		**DINNER**		**BEDTIME**	
	BEFORE	AFTER	BEFORE	AFTER	BEFORE	AFTER	BEFORE	AFTER
BLOOD SUGAR								
BLOOD PRESSURE								
Date __/__/__ **Thursday**	**BREAKFAST**		**LUNCH**		**DINNER**		**BEDTIME**	
	BEFORE	AFTER	BEFORE	AFTER	BEFORE	AFTER	BEFORE	AFTER
BLOOD SUGAR								
BLOOD PRESSURE								
Date __/__/__ **Friday**	**BREAKFAST**		**LUNCH**		**DINNER**		**BEDTIME**	
	BEFORE	AFTER	BEFORE	AFTER	BEFORE	AFTER	BEFORE	AFTER
BLOOD SUGAR								
BLOOD PRESSURE								
Date __/__/__ **Saturday**	**BREAKFAST**		**LUNCH**		**DINNER**		**BEDTIME**	
	BEFORE	AFTER	BEFORE	AFTER	BEFORE	AFTER	BEFORE	AFTER
BLOOD SUGAR								
BLOOD PRESSURE								
Date __/__/__ **Sunday**	**BREAKFAST**		**LUNCH**		**DINNER**		**BEDTIME**	
	BEFORE	AFTER	BEFORE	AFTER	BEFORE	AFTER	BEFORE	AFTER
BLOOD SUGAR								
BLOOD PRESSURE								

NOTES: _____
_____
_____
_____

Month: _____ **Week Commencing:** _____

Date __/__/__ Monday	BREAKFAST		LUNCH		DINNER		BEDTIME	
	BEFORE	AFTER	BEFORE	AFTER	BEFORE	AFTER	BEFORE	AFTER
BLOOD SUGAR								
BLOOD PRESSURE								

Date __/__/__ Tuesday	BREAKFAST		LUNCH		DINNER		BEDTIME	
	BEFORE	AFTER	BEFORE	AFTER	BEFORE	AFTER	BEFORE	AFTER
BLOOD SUGAR								
BLOOD PRESSURE								

Date __/__/__ Wednesday	BREAKFAST		LUNCH		DINNER		BEDTIME	
	BEFORE	AFTER	BEFORE	AFTER	BEFORE	AFTER	BEFORE	AFTER
BLOOD SUGAR								
BLOOD PRESSURE								

Date __/__/__ Thursday	BREAKFAST		LUNCH		DINNER		BEDTIME	
	BEFORE	AFTER	BEFORE	AFTER	BEFORE	AFTER	BEFORE	AFTER
BLOOD SUGAR								
BLOOD PRESSURE								

Date __/__/__ Friday	BREAKFAST		LUNCH		DINNER		BEDTIME	
	BEFORE	AFTER	BEFORE	AFTER	BEFORE	AFTER	BEFORE	AFTER
BLOOD SUGAR								
BLOOD PRESSURE								

Date __/__/__ Saturday	BREAKFAST		LUNCH		DINNER		BEDTIME	
	BEFORE	AFTER	BEFORE	AFTER	BEFORE	AFTER	BEFORE	AFTER
BLOOD SUGAR								
BLOOD PRESSURE								

Date __/__/__ Sunday	BREAKFAST		LUNCH		DINNER		BEDTIME	
	BEFORE	AFTER	BEFORE	AFTER	BEFORE	AFTER	BEFORE	AFTER
BLOOD SUGAR								
BLOOD PRESSURE								

NOTES: _____

_____

_____

Month: _____ **Week Commencing:** _____

Date __/__/__	BREAKFAST		LUNCH		DINNER		BEDTIME	
Monday	BEFORE	AFTER	BEFORE	AFTER	BEFORE	AFTER	BEFORE	AFTER
BLOOD SUGAR								
BLOOD PRESSURE								
Date __/__/__	BREAKFAST		LUNCH		DINNER		BEDTIME	
Tuesday	BEFORE	AFTER	BEFORE	AFTER	BEFORE	AFTER	BEFORE	AFTER
BLOOD SUGAR								
BLOOD PRESSURE								
Date __/__/__	BREAKFAST		LUNCH		DINNER		BEDTIME	
Wednesday	BEFORE	AFTER	BEFORE	AFTER	BEFORE	AFTER	BEFORE	AFTER
BLOOD SUGAR								
BLOOD PRESSURE								
Date __/__/__	BREAKFAST		LUNCH		DINNER		BEDTIME	
Thursday	BEFORE	AFTER	BEFORE	AFTER	BEFORE	AFTER	BEFORE	AFTER
BLOOD SUGAR								
BLOOD PRESSURE								
Date __/__/__	BREAKFAST		LUNCH		DINNER		BEDTIME	
Friday	BEFORE	AFTER	BEFORE	AFTER	BEFORE	AFTER	BEFORE	AFTER
BLOOD SUGAR								
BLOOD PRESSURE								
Date __/__/__	BREAKFAST		LUNCH		DINNER		BEDTIME	
Saturday	BEFORE	AFTER	BEFORE	AFTER	BEFORE	AFTER	BEFORE	AFTER
BLOOD SUGAR								
BLOOD PRESSURE								
Date __/__/__	BREAKFAST		LUNCH		DINNER		BEDTIME	
Sunday	BEFORE	AFTER	BEFORE	AFTER	BEFORE	AFTER	BEFORE	AFTER
BLOOD SUGAR								
BLOOD PRESSURE								

NOTES: _____
_____
_____
_____

Month: _____ **Week Commencing:** _____

Date __/__/__	BREAKFAST		LUNCH		DINNER		BEDTIME	
Monday	BEFORE	AFTER	BEFORE	AFTER	BEFORE	AFTER	BEFORE	AFTER
BLOOD SUGAR								
BLOOD PRESSURE								

Date __/__/__	BREAKFAST		LUNCH		DINNER		BEDTIME	
Tuesday	BEFORE	AFTER	BEFORE	AFTER	BEFORE	AFTER	BEFORE	AFTER
BLOOD SUGAR								
BLOOD PRESSURE								

Date __/__/__	BREAKFAST		LUNCH		DINNER		BEDTIME	
Wednesday	BEFORE	AFTER	BEFORE	AFTER	BEFORE	AFTER	BEFORE	AFTER
BLOOD SUGAR								
BLOOD PRESSURE								

Date __/__/__	BREAKFAST		LUNCH		DINNER		BEDTIME	
Thursday	BEFORE	AFTER	BEFORE	AFTER	BEFORE	AFTER	BEFORE	AFTER
BLOOD SUGAR								
BLOOD PRESSURE								

Date __/__/__	BREAKFAST		LUNCH		DINNER		BEDTIME	
Friday	BEFORE	AFTER	BEFORE	AFTER	BEFORE	AFTER	BEFORE	AFTER
BLOOD SUGAR								
BLOOD PRESSURE								

Date __/__/__	BREAKFAST		LUNCH		DINNER		BEDTIME	
Saturday	BEFORE	AFTER	BEFORE	AFTER	BEFORE	AFTER	BEFORE	AFTER
BLOOD SUGAR								
BLOOD PRESSURE								

Date __/__/__	BREAKFAST		LUNCH		DINNER		BEDTIME	
Sunday	BEFORE	AFTER	BEFORE	AFTER	BEFORE	AFTER	BEFORE	AFTER
BLOOD SUGAR								
BLOOD PRESSURE								

NOTES: _____

_____

_____

Month: _____ **Week Commencing:** _____

Date __/__/__	BREAKFAST		LUNCH		DINNER		BEDTIME	
Monday	BEFORE	AFTER	BEFORE	AFTER	BEFORE	AFTER	BEFORE	AFTER
BLOOD SUGAR								
BLOOD PRESSURE								
Date __/__/__	BREAKFAST		LUNCH		DINNER		BEDTIME	
Tuesday	BEFORE	AFTER	BEFORE	AFTER	BEFORE	AFTER	BEFORE	AFTER
BLOOD SUGAR								
BLOOD PRESSURE								
Date __/__/__	BREAKFAST		LUNCH		DINNER		BEDTIME	
Wednesday	BEFORE	AFTER	BEFORE	AFTER	BEFORE	AFTER	BEFORE	AFTER
BLOOD SUGAR								
BLOOD PRESSURE								
Date __/__/__	BREAKFAST		LUNCH		DINNER		BEDTIME	
Thursday	BEFORE	AFTER	BEFORE	AFTER	BEFORE	AFTER	BEFORE	AFTER
BLOOD SUGAR								
BLOOD PRESSURE								
Date __/__/__	BREAKFAST		LUNCH		DINNER		BEDTIME	
Friday	BEFORE	AFTER	BEFORE	AFTER	BEFORE	AFTER	BEFORE	AFTER
BLOOD SUGAR								
BLOOD PRESSURE								
Date __/__/__	BREAKFAST		LUNCH		DINNER		BEDTIME	
Saturday	BEFORE	AFTER	BEFORE	AFTER	BEFORE	AFTER	BEFORE	AFTER
BLOOD SUGAR								
BLOOD PRESSURE								
Date __/__/__	BREAKFAST		LUNCH		DINNER		BEDTIME	
Sunday	BEFORE	AFTER	BEFORE	AFTER	BEFORE	AFTER	BEFORE	AFTER
BLOOD SUGAR								
BLOOD PRESSURE								

NOTES: _____
_____
_____
_____

Month: _____ **Week Commencing:** _____

Date __/__/__	BREAKFAST		LUNCH		DINNER		BEDTIME	
Monday	BEFORE	AFTER	BEFORE	AFTER	BEFORE	AFTER	BEFORE	AFTER
BLOOD SUGAR								
BLOOD PRESSURE								

Date __/__/__	BREAKFAST		LUNCH		DINNER		BEDTIME	
Tuesday	BEFORE	AFTER	BEFORE	AFTER	BEFORE	AFTER	BEFORE	AFTER
BLOOD SUGAR								
BLOOD PRESSURE								

Date __/__/__	BREAKFAST		LUNCH		DINNER		BEDTIME	
Wednesday	BEFORE	AFTER	BEFORE	AFTER	BEFORE	AFTER	BEFORE	AFTER
BLOOD SUGAR								
BLOOD PRESSURE								

Date __/__/__	BREAKFAST		LUNCH		DINNER		BEDTIME	
Thursday	BEFORE	AFTER	BEFORE	AFTER	BEFORE	AFTER	BEFORE	AFTER
BLOOD SUGAR								
BLOOD PRESSURE								

Date __/__/__	BREAKFAST		LUNCH		DINNER		BEDTIME	
Friday	BEFORE	AFTER	BEFORE	AFTER	BEFORE	AFTER	BEFORE	AFTER
BLOOD SUGAR								
BLOOD PRESSURE								

Date __/__/__	BREAKFAST		LUNCH		DINNER		BEDTIME	
Saturday	BEFORE	AFTER	BEFORE	AFTER	BEFORE	AFTER	BEFORE	AFTER
BLOOD SUGAR								
BLOOD PRESSURE								

Date __/__/__	BREAKFAST		LUNCH		DINNER		BEDTIME	
Sunday	BEFORE	AFTER	BEFORE	AFTER	BEFORE	AFTER	BEFORE	AFTER
BLOOD SUGAR								
BLOOD PRESSURE								

NOTES: _____

_____

_____

Month: _____ **Week Commencing:** _____

Date __/__/__	BREAKFAST		LUNCH		DINNER		BEDTIME	
Monday	BEFORE	AFTER	BEFORE	AFTER	BEFORE	AFTER	BEFORE	AFTER
BLOOD SUGAR								
BLOOD PRESSURE								
Date __/__/__	BREAKFAST		LUNCH		DINNER		BEDTIME	
Tuesday	BEFORE	AFTER	BEFORE	AFTER	BEFORE	AFTER	BEFORE	AFTER
BLOOD SUGAR								
BLOOD PRESSURE								
Date __/__/__	BREAKFAST		LUNCH		DINNER		BEDTIME	
Wednesday	BEFORE	AFTER	BEFORE	AFTER	BEFORE	AFTER	BEFORE	AFTER
BLOOD SUGAR								
BLOOD PRESSURE								
Date __/__/__	BREAKFAST		LUNCH		DINNER		BEDTIME	
Thursday	BEFORE	AFTER	BEFORE	AFTER	BEFORE	AFTER	BEFORE	AFTER
BLOOD SUGAR								
BLOOD PRESSURE								
Date __/__/__	BREAKFAST		LUNCH		DINNER		BEDTIME	
Friday	BEFORE	AFTER	BEFORE	AFTER	BEFORE	AFTER	BEFORE	AFTER
BLOOD SUGAR								
BLOOD PRESSURE								
Date __/__/__	BREAKFAST		LUNCH		DINNER		BEDTIME	
Saturday	BEFORE	AFTER	BEFORE	AFTER	BEFORE	AFTER	BEFORE	AFTER
BLOOD SUGAR								
BLOOD PRESSURE								
Date __/__/__	BREAKFAST		LUNCH		DINNER		BEDTIME	
Sunday	BEFORE	AFTER	BEFORE	AFTER	BEFORE	AFTER	BEFORE	AFTER
BLOOD SUGAR								
BLOOD PRESSURE								

NOTES: _____
_____
_____
_____

Month: _____ **Week Commencing:** _____

Date ___/___/___	BREAKFAST		LUNCH		DINNER		BEDTIME	
Monday	BEFORE	AFTER	BEFORE	AFTER	BEFORE	AFTER	BEFORE	AFTER
BLOOD SUGAR								
BLOOD PRESSURE								

Date ___/___/___	BREAKFAST		LUNCH		DINNER		BEDTIME	
Tuesday	BEFORE	AFTER	BEFORE	AFTER	BEFORE	AFTER	BEFORE	AFTER
BLOOD SUGAR								
BLOOD PRESSURE								

Date ___/___/___	BREAKFAST		LUNCH		DINNER		BEDTIME	
Wednesday	BEFORE	AFTER	BEFORE	AFTER	BEFORE	AFTER	BEFORE	AFTER
BLOOD SUGAR								
BLOOD PRESSURE								

Date ___/___/___	BREAKFAST		LUNCH		DINNER		BEDTIME	
Thursday	BEFORE	AFTER	BEFORE	AFTER	BEFORE	AFTER	BEFORE	AFTER
BLOOD SUGAR								
BLOOD PRESSURE								

Date ___/___/___	BREAKFAST		LUNCH		DINNER		BEDTIME	
Friday	BEFORE	AFTER	BEFORE	AFTER	BEFORE	AFTER	BEFORE	AFTER
BLOOD SUGAR								
BLOOD PRESSURE								

Date ___/___/___	BREAKFAST		LUNCH		DINNER		BEDTIME	
Saturday	BEFORE	AFTER	BEFORE	AFTER	BEFORE	AFTER	BEFORE	AFTER
BLOOD SUGAR								
BLOOD PRESSURE								

Date ___/___/___	BREAKFAST		LUNCH		DINNER		BEDTIME	
Sunday	BEFORE	AFTER	BEFORE	AFTER	BEFORE	AFTER	BEFORE	AFTER
BLOOD SUGAR								
BLOOD PRESSURE								

NOTES: _____
_____
_____
_____

Month: _____ **Week Commencing:** _____

Date __/__/__	BREAKFAST		LUNCH		DINNER		BEDTIME	
Monday	BEFORE	AFTER	BEFORE	AFTER	BEFORE	AFTER	BEFORE	AFTER
BLOOD SUGAR								
BLOOD PRESSURE								
Date __/__/__	BREAKFAST		LUNCH		DINNER		BEDTIME	
Tuesday	BEFORE	AFTER	BEFORE	AFTER	BEFORE	AFTER	BEFORE	AFTER
BLOOD SUGAR								
BLOOD PRESSURE								
Date __/__/__	BREAKFAST		LUNCH		DINNER		BEDTIME	
Wednesday	BEFORE	AFTER	BEFORE	AFTER	BEFORE	AFTER	BEFORE	AFTER
BLOOD SUGAR								
BLOOD PRESSURE								
Date __/__/__	BREAKFAST		LUNCH		DINNER		BEDTIME	
Thursday	BEFORE	AFTER	BEFORE	AFTER	BEFORE	AFTER	BEFORE	AFTER
BLOOD SUGAR								
BLOOD PRESSURE								
Date __/__/__	BREAKFAST		LUNCH		DINNER		BEDTIME	
Friday	BEFORE	AFTER	BEFORE	AFTER	BEFORE	AFTER	BEFORE	AFTER
BLOOD SUGAR								
BLOOD PRESSURE								
Date __/__/__	BREAKFAST		LUNCH		DINNER		BEDTIME	
Saturday	BEFORE	AFTER	BEFORE	AFTER	BEFORE	AFTER	BEFORE	AFTER
BLOOD SUGAR								
BLOOD PRESSURE								
Date __/__/__	BREAKFAST		LUNCH		DINNER		BEDTIME	
Sunday	BEFORE	AFTER	BEFORE	AFTER	BEFORE	AFTER	BEFORE	AFTER
BLOOD SUGAR								
BLOOD PRESSURE								

NOTES: _____
_____
_____
_____

Month: _____ Week Commencing: _____

Date __/__/__	BREAKFAST		LUNCH		DINNER		BEDTIME	
Monday	BEFORE	AFTER	BEFORE	AFTER	BEFORE	AFTER	BEFORE	AFTER
BLOOD SUGAR								
BLOOD PRESSURE								
Date __/__/__	BREAKFAST		LUNCH		DINNER		BEDTIME	
Tuesday	BEFORE	AFTER	BEFORE	AFTER	BEFORE	AFTER	BEFORE	AFTER
BLOOD SUGAR								
BLOOD PRESSURE								
Date __/__/__	BREAKFAST		LUNCH		DINNER		BEDTIME	
Wednesday	BEFORE	AFTER	BEFORE	AFTER	BEFORE	AFTER	BEFORE	AFTER
BLOOD SUGAR								
BLOOD PRESSURE								
Date __/__/__	BREAKFAST		LUNCH		DINNER		BEDTIME	
Thursday	BEFORE	AFTER	BEFORE	AFTER	BEFORE	AFTER	BEFORE	AFTER
BLOOD SUGAR								
BLOOD PRESSURE								
Date __/__/__	BREAKFAST		LUNCH		DINNER		BEDTIME	
Friday	BEFORE	AFTER	BEFORE	AFTER	BEFORE	AFTER	BEFORE	AFTER
BLOOD SUGAR								
BLOOD PRESSURE								
Date __/__/__	BREAKFAST		LUNCH		DINNER		BEDTIME	
Saturday	BEFORE	AFTER	BEFORE	AFTER	BEFORE	AFTER	BEFORE	AFTER
BLOOD SUGAR								
BLOOD PRESSURE								
Date __/__/__	BREAKFAST		LUNCH		DINNER		BEDTIME	
Sunday	BEFORE	AFTER	BEFORE	AFTER	BEFORE	AFTER	BEFORE	AFTER
BLOOD SUGAR								
BLOOD PRESSURE								

NOTES: _____
_____
_____
_____

Month: _____ **Week Commencing:** _____

Date __/__/__	BREAKFAST		LUNCH		DINNER		BEDTIME	
Monday	BEFORE	AFTER	BEFORE	AFTER	BEFORE	AFTER	BEFORE	AFTER
BLOOD SUGAR								
BLOOD PRESSURE								
Date __/__/__	BREAKFAST		LUNCH		DINNER		BEDTIME	
Tuesday	BEFORE	AFTER	BEFORE	AFTER	BEFORE	AFTER	BEFORE	AFTER
BLOOD SUGAR								
BLOOD PRESSURE								
Date __/__/__	BREAKFAST		LUNCH		DINNER		BEDTIME	
Wednesday	BEFORE	AFTER	BEFORE	AFTER	BEFORE	AFTER	BEFORE	AFTER
BLOOD SUGAR								
BLOOD PRESSURE								
Date __/__/__	BREAKFAST		LUNCH		DINNER		BEDTIME	
Thursday	BEFORE	AFTER	BEFORE	AFTER	BEFORE	AFTER	BEFORE	AFTER
BLOOD SUGAR								
BLOOD PRESSURE								
Date __/__/__	BREAKFAST		LUNCH		DINNER		BEDTIME	
Friday	BEFORE	AFTER	BEFORE	AFTER	BEFORE	AFTER	BEFORE	AFTER
BLOOD SUGAR								
BLOOD PRESSURE								
Date __/__/__	BREAKFAST		LUNCH		DINNER		BEDTIME	
Saturday	BEFORE	AFTER	BEFORE	AFTER	BEFORE	AFTER	BEFORE	AFTER
BLOOD SUGAR								
BLOOD PRESSURE								
Date __/__/__	BREAKFAST		LUNCH		DINNER		BEDTIME	
Sunday	BEFORE	AFTER	BEFORE	AFTER	BEFORE	AFTER	BEFORE	AFTER
BLOOD SUGAR								
BLOOD PRESSURE								

NOTES: _____
_____
_____
_____

Month: _____ **Week Commencing:** _____

Date __/__/__	BREAKFAST		LUNCH		DINNER		BEDTIME	
Monday	BEFORE	AFTER	BEFORE	AFTER	BEFORE	AFTER	BEFORE	AFTER
BLOOD SUGAR								
BLOOD PRESSURE								
Date __/__/__	BREAKFAST		LUNCH		DINNER		BEDTIME	
Tuesday	BEFORE	AFTER	BEFORE	AFTER	BEFORE	AFTER	BEFORE	AFTER
BLOOD SUGAR								
BLOOD PRESSURE								
Date __/__/__	BREAKFAST		LUNCH		DINNER		BEDTIME	
Wednesday	BEFORE	AFTER	BEFORE	AFTER	BEFORE	AFTER	BEFORE	AFTER
BLOOD SUGAR								
BLOOD PRESSURE								
Date __/__/__	BREAKFAST		LUNCH		DINNER		BEDTIME	
Thursday	BEFORE	AFTER	BEFORE	AFTER	BEFORE	AFTER	BEFORE	AFTER
BLOOD SUGAR								
BLOOD PRESSURE								
Date __/__/__	BREAKFAST		LUNCH		DINNER		BEDTIME	
Friday	BEFORE	AFTER	BEFORE	AFTER	BEFORE	AFTER	BEFORE	AFTER
BLOOD SUGAR								
BLOOD PRESSURE								
Date __/__/__	BREAKFAST		LUNCH		DINNER		BEDTIME	
Saturday	BEFORE	AFTER	BEFORE	AFTER	BEFORE	AFTER	BEFORE	AFTER
BLOOD SUGAR								
BLOOD PRESSURE								
Date __/__/__	BREAKFAST		LUNCH		DINNER		BEDTIME	
Sunday	BEFORE	AFTER	BEFORE	AFTER	BEFORE	AFTER	BEFORE	AFTER
BLOOD SUGAR								
BLOOD PRESSURE								

NOTES: _____
_____
_____
_____

Month: _____ Week Commencing: _____

Date __/__/__ Monday	BREAKFAST		LUNCH		DINNER		BEDTIME	
	BEFORE	AFTER	BEFORE	AFTER	BEFORE	AFTER	BEFORE	AFTER
BLOOD SUGAR								
BLOOD PRESSURE								

Date __/__/__ Tuesday	BREAKFAST		LUNCH		DINNER		BEDTIME	
	BEFORE	AFTER	BEFORE	AFTER	BEFORE	AFTER	BEFORE	AFTER
BLOOD SUGAR								
BLOOD PRESSURE								

Date __/__/__ Wednesday	BREAKFAST		LUNCH		DINNER		BEDTIME	
	BEFORE	AFTER	BEFORE	AFTER	BEFORE	AFTER	BEFORE	AFTER
BLOOD SUGAR								
BLOOD PRESSURE								

Date __/__/__ Thursday	BREAKFAST		LUNCH		DINNER		BEDTIME	
	BEFORE	AFTER	BEFORE	AFTER	BEFORE	AFTER	BEFORE	AFTER
BLOOD SUGAR								
BLOOD PRESSURE								

Date __/__/__ Friday	BREAKFAST		LUNCH		DINNER		BEDTIME	
	BEFORE	AFTER	BEFORE	AFTER	BEFORE	AFTER	BEFORE	AFTER
BLOOD SUGAR								
BLOOD PRESSURE								

Date __/__/__ Saturday	BREAKFAST		LUNCH		DINNER		BEDTIME	
	BEFORE	AFTER	BEFORE	AFTER	BEFORE	AFTER	BEFORE	AFTER
BLOOD SUGAR								
BLOOD PRESSURE								

Date __/__/__ Sunday	BREAKFAST		LUNCH		DINNER		BEDTIME	
	BEFORE	AFTER	BEFORE	AFTER	BEFORE	AFTER	BEFORE	AFTER
BLOOD SUGAR								
BLOOD PRESSURE								

NOTES: _____

_____

_____

_____

Month: _____ **Week Commencing:** _____

Date __/__/__	BREAKFAST		LUNCH		DINNER		BEDTIME	
Monday	BEFORE	AFTER	BEFORE	AFTER	BEFORE	AFTER	BEFORE	AFTER
BLOOD SUGAR								
BLOOD PRESSURE								
Date __/__/__	BREAKFAST		LUNCH		DINNER		BEDTIME	
Tuesday	BEFORE	AFTER	BEFORE	AFTER	BEFORE	AFTER	BEFORE	AFTER
BLOOD SUGAR								
BLOOD PRESSURE								
Date __/__/__	BREAKFAST		LUNCH		DINNER		BEDTIME	
Wednesday	BEFORE	AFTER	BEFORE	AFTER	BEFORE	AFTER	BEFORE	AFTER
BLOOD SUGAR								
BLOOD PRESSURE								
Date __/__/__	BREAKFAST		LUNCH		DINNER		BEDTIME	
Thursday	BEFORE	AFTER	BEFORE	AFTER	BEFORE	AFTER	BEFORE	AFTER
BLOOD SUGAR								
BLOOD PRESSURE								
Date __/__/__	BREAKFAST		LUNCH		DINNER		BEDTIME	
Friday	BEFORE	AFTER	BEFORE	AFTER	BEFORE	AFTER	BEFORE	AFTER
BLOOD SUGAR								
BLOOD PRESSURE								
Date __/__/__	BREAKFAST		LUNCH		DINNER		BEDTIME	
Saturday	BEFORE	AFTER	BEFORE	AFTER	BEFORE	AFTER	BEFORE	AFTER
BLOOD SUGAR								
BLOOD PRESSURE								
Date __/__/__	BREAKFAST		LUNCH		DINNER		BEDTIME	
Sunday	BEFORE	AFTER	BEFORE	AFTER	BEFORE	AFTER	BEFORE	AFTER
BLOOD SUGAR								
BLOOD PRESSURE								

NOTES: _____

_____

_____

_____

Month: _____ Week Commencing: _____

Date __/__/__	BREAKFAST		LUNCH		DINNER		BEDTIME	
Monday	BEFORE	AFTER	BEFORE	AFTER	BEFORE	AFTER	BEFORE	AFTER
BLOOD SUGAR								
BLOOD PRESSURE								

Date __/__/__	BREAKFAST		LUNCH		DINNER		BEDTIME	
Tuesday	BEFORE	AFTER	BEFORE	AFTER	BEFORE	AFTER	BEFORE	AFTER
BLOOD SUGAR								
BLOOD PRESSURE								

Date __/__/__	BREAKFAST		LUNCH		DINNER		BEDTIME	
Wednesday	BEFORE	AFTER	BEFORE	AFTER	BEFORE	AFTER	BEFORE	AFTER
BLOOD SUGAR								
BLOOD PRESSURE								

Date __/__/__	BREAKFAST		LUNCH		DINNER		BEDTIME	
Thursday	BEFORE	AFTER	BEFORE	AFTER	BEFORE	AFTER	BEFORE	AFTER
BLOOD SUGAR								
BLOOD PRESSURE								

Date __/__/__	BREAKFAST		LUNCH		DINNER		BEDTIME	
Friday	BEFORE	AFTER	BEFORE	AFTER	BEFORE	AFTER	BEFORE	AFTER
BLOOD SUGAR								
BLOOD PRESSURE								

Date __/__/__	BREAKFAST		LUNCH		DINNER		BEDTIME	
Saturday	BEFORE	AFTER	BEFORE	AFTER	BEFORE	AFTER	BEFORE	AFTER
BLOOD SUGAR								
BLOOD PRESSURE								

Date __/__/__	BREAKFAST		LUNCH		DINNER		BEDTIME	
Sunday	BEFORE	AFTER	BEFORE	AFTER	BEFORE	AFTER	BEFORE	AFTER
BLOOD SUGAR								
BLOOD PRESSURE								

NOTES: _____
_____
_____
_____

Month: _____ **Week Commencing:** _____

Date __/__/__	BREAKFAST		LUNCH		DINNER		BEDTIME	
Monday	BEFORE	AFTER	BEFORE	AFTER	BEFORE	AFTER	BEFORE	AFTER
BLOOD SUGAR								
BLOOD PRESSURE								
Date __/__/__	BREAKFAST		LUNCH		DINNER		BEDTIME	
Tuesday	BEFORE	AFTER	BEFORE	AFTER	BEFORE	AFTER	BEFORE	AFTER
BLOOD SUGAR								
BLOOD PRESSURE								
Date __/__/__	BREAKFAST		LUNCH		DINNER		BEDTIME	
Wednesday	BEFORE	AFTER	BEFORE	AFTER	BEFORE	AFTER	BEFORE	AFTER
BLOOD SUGAR								
BLOOD PRESSURE								
Date __/__/__	BREAKFAST		LUNCH		DINNER		BEDTIME	
Thursday	BEFORE	AFTER	BEFORE	AFTER	BEFORE	AFTER	BEFORE	AFTER
BLOOD SUGAR								
BLOOD PRESSURE								
Date __/__/__	BREAKFAST		LUNCH		DINNER		BEDTIME	
Friday	BEFORE	AFTER	BEFORE	AFTER	BEFORE	AFTER	BEFORE	AFTER
BLOOD SUGAR								
BLOOD PRESSURE								
Date __/__/__	BREAKFAST		LUNCH		DINNER		BEDTIME	
Saturday	BEFORE	AFTER	BEFORE	AFTER	BEFORE	AFTER	BEFORE	AFTER
BLOOD SUGAR								
BLOOD PRESSURE								
Date __/__/__	BREAKFAST		LUNCH		DINNER		BEDTIME	
Sunday	BEFORE	AFTER	BEFORE	AFTER	BEFORE	AFTER	BEFORE	AFTER
BLOOD SUGAR								
BLOOD PRESSURE								

NOTES: _____
_____
_____

Month: _____ **Week Commencing:** _____

Date __/__/__	BREAKFAST		LUNCH		DINNER		BEDTIME	
Monday	BEFORE	AFTER	BEFORE	AFTER	BEFORE	AFTER	BEFORE	AFTER
BLOOD SUGAR								
BLOOD PRESSURE								
Date __/__/__	BREAKFAST		LUNCH		DINNER		BEDTIME	
Tuesday	BEFORE	AFTER	BEFORE	AFTER	BEFORE	AFTER	BEFORE	AFTER
BLOOD SUGAR								
BLOOD PRESSURE								
Date __/__/__	BREAKFAST		LUNCH		DINNER		BEDTIME	
Wednesday	BEFORE	AFTER	BEFORE	AFTER	BEFORE	AFTER	BEFORE	AFTER
BLOOD SUGAR								
BLOOD PRESSURE								
Date __/__/__	BREAKFAST		LUNCH		DINNER		BEDTIME	
Thursday	BEFORE	AFTER	BEFORE	AFTER	BEFORE	AFTER	BEFORE	AFTER
BLOOD SUGAR								
BLOOD PRESSURE								
Date __/__/__	BREAKFAST		LUNCH		DINNER		BEDTIME	
Friday	BEFORE	AFTER	BEFORE	AFTER	BEFORE	AFTER	BEFORE	AFTER
BLOOD SUGAR								
BLOOD PRESSURE								
Date __/__/__	BREAKFAST		LUNCH		DINNER		BEDTIME	
Saturday	BEFORE	AFTER	BEFORE	AFTER	BEFORE	AFTER	BEFORE	AFTER
BLOOD SUGAR								
BLOOD PRESSURE								
Date __/__/__	BREAKFAST		LUNCH		DINNER		BEDTIME	
Sunday	BEFORE	AFTER	BEFORE	AFTER	BEFORE	AFTER	BEFORE	AFTER
BLOOD SUGAR								
BLOOD PRESSURE								

NOTES: _____
_____
_____
_____

Month: _____ **Week Commencing:** _____

Date __/__/__	BREAKFAST		LUNCH		DINNER		BEDTIME	
Monday	BEFORE	AFTER	BEFORE	AFTER	BEFORE	AFTER	BEFORE	AFTER
BLOOD SUGAR								
BLOOD PRESSURE								
Date __/__/__	BREAKFAST		LUNCH		DINNER		BEDTIME	
Tuesday	BEFORE	AFTER	BEFORE	AFTER	BEFORE	AFTER	BEFORE	AFTER
BLOOD SUGAR								
BLOOD PRESSURE								
Date __/__/__	BREAKFAST		LUNCH		DINNER		BEDTIME	
Wednesday	BEFORE	AFTER	BEFORE	AFTER	BEFORE	AFTER	BEFORE	AFTER
BLOOD SUGAR								
BLOOD PRESSURE								
Date __/__/__	BREAKFAST		LUNCH		DINNER		BEDTIME	
Thursday	BEFORE	AFTER	BEFORE	AFTER	BEFORE	AFTER	BEFORE	AFTER
BLOOD SUGAR								
BLOOD PRESSURE								
Date __/__/__	BREAKFAST		LUNCH		DINNER		BEDTIME	
Friday	BEFORE	AFTER	BEFORE	AFTER	BEFORE	AFTER	BEFORE	AFTER
BLOOD SUGAR								
BLOOD PRESSURE								
Date __/__/__	BREAKFAST		LUNCH		DINNER		BEDTIME	
Saturday	BEFORE	AFTER	BEFORE	AFTER	BEFORE	AFTER	BEFORE	AFTER
BLOOD SUGAR								
BLOOD PRESSURE								
Date __/__/__	BREAKFAST		LUNCH		DINNER		BEDTIME	
Sunday	BEFORE	AFTER	BEFORE	AFTER	BEFORE	AFTER	BEFORE	AFTER
BLOOD SUGAR								
BLOOD PRESSURE								

NOTES: _____

_____

_____

Month: _____ Week Commencing: _____

Date __/__/__	BREAKFAST		LUNCH		DINNER		BEDTIME	
Monday	BEFORE	AFTER	BEFORE	AFTER	BEFORE	AFTER	BEFORE	AFTER
BLOOD SUGAR								
BLOOD PRESSURE								
Date __/__/__	BREAKFAST		LUNCH		DINNER		BEDTIME	
Tuesday	BEFORE	AFTER	BEFORE	AFTER	BEFORE	AFTER	BEFORE	AFTER
BLOOD SUGAR								
BLOOD PRESSURE								
Date __/__/__	BREAKFAST		LUNCH		DINNER		BEDTIME	
Wednesday	BEFORE	AFTER	BEFORE	AFTER	BEFORE	AFTER	BEFORE	AFTER
BLOOD SUGAR								
BLOOD PRESSURE								
Date __/__/__	BREAKFAST		LUNCH		DINNER		BEDTIME	
Thursday	BEFORE	AFTER	BEFORE	AFTER	BEFORE	AFTER	BEFORE	AFTER
BLOOD SUGAR								
BLOOD PRESSURE								
Date __/__/__	BREAKFAST		LUNCH		DINNER		BEDTIME	
Friday	BEFORE	AFTER	BEFORE	AFTER	BEFORE	AFTER	BEFORE	AFTER
BLOOD SUGAR								
BLOOD PRESSURE								
Date __/__/__	BREAKFAST		LUNCH		DINNER		BEDTIME	
Saturday	BEFORE	AFTER	BEFORE	AFTER	BEFORE	AFTER	BEFORE	AFTER
BLOOD SUGAR								
BLOOD PRESSURE								
Date __/__/__	BREAKFAST		LUNCH		DINNER		BEDTIME	
Sunday	BEFORE	AFTER	BEFORE	AFTER	BEFORE	AFTER	BEFORE	AFTER
BLOOD SUGAR								
BLOOD PRESSURE								

NOTES: _____
_____
_____
_____

Month: _____ **Week Commencing:** _____

Date __/__/__	BREAKFAST		LUNCH		DINNER		BEDTIME	
Monday	BEFORE	AFTER	BEFORE	AFTER	BEFORE	AFTER	BEFORE	AFTER
BLOOD SUGAR								
BLOOD PRESSURE								

Date __/__/__	BREAKFAST		LUNCH		DINNER		BEDTIME	
Tuesday	BEFORE	AFTER	BEFORE	AFTER	BEFORE	AFTER	BEFORE	AFTER
BLOOD SUGAR								
BLOOD PRESSURE								

Date __/__/__	BREAKFAST		LUNCH		DINNER		BEDTIME	
Wednesday	BEFORE	AFTER	BEFORE	AFTER	BEFORE	AFTER	BEFORE	AFTER
BLOOD SUGAR								
BLOOD PRESSURE								

Date __/__/__	BREAKFAST		LUNCH		DINNER		BEDTIME	
Thursday	BEFORE	AFTER	BEFORE	AFTER	BEFORE	AFTER	BEFORE	AFTER
BLOOD SUGAR								
BLOOD PRESSURE								

Date __/__/__	BREAKFAST		LUNCH		DINNER		BEDTIME	
Friday	BEFORE	AFTER	BEFORE	AFTER	BEFORE	AFTER	BEFORE	AFTER
BLOOD SUGAR								
BLOOD PRESSURE								

Date __/__/__	BREAKFAST		LUNCH		DINNER		BEDTIME	
Saturday	BEFORE	AFTER	BEFORE	AFTER	BEFORE	AFTER	BEFORE	AFTER
BLOOD SUGAR								
BLOOD PRESSURE								

Date __/__/__	BREAKFAST		LUNCH		DINNER		BEDTIME	
Sunday	BEFORE	AFTER	BEFORE	AFTER	BEFORE	AFTER	BEFORE	AFTER
BLOOD SUGAR								
BLOOD PRESSURE								

NOTES: _____

_____

_____

_____

Month: _____ **Week Commencing:** _____

Date __/__/__ Monday	BREAKFAST		LUNCH		DINNER		BEDTIME	
	BEFORE	AFTER	BEFORE	AFTER	BEFORE	AFTER	BEFORE	AFTER
BLOOD SUGAR								
BLOOD PRESSURE								

Date __/__/__ Tuesday	BREAKFAST		LUNCH		DINNER		BEDTIME	
	BEFORE	AFTER	BEFORE	AFTER	BEFORE	AFTER	BEFORE	AFTER
BLOOD SUGAR								
BLOOD PRESSURE								

Date __/__/__ Wednesday	BREAKFAST		LUNCH		DINNER		BEDTIME	
	BEFORE	AFTER	BEFORE	AFTER	BEFORE	AFTER	BEFORE	AFTER
BLOOD SUGAR								
BLOOD PRESSURE								

Date __/__/__ Thursday	BREAKFAST		LUNCH		DINNER		BEDTIME	
	BEFORE	AFTER	BEFORE	AFTER	BEFORE	AFTER	BEFORE	AFTER
BLOOD SUGAR								
BLOOD PRESSURE								

Date __/__/__ Friday	BREAKFAST		LUNCH		DINNER		BEDTIME	
	BEFORE	AFTER	BEFORE	AFTER	BEFORE	AFTER	BEFORE	AFTER
BLOOD SUGAR								
BLOOD PRESSURE								

Date __/__/__ Saturday	BREAKFAST		LUNCH		DINNER		BEDTIME	
	BEFORE	AFTER	BEFORE	AFTER	BEFORE	AFTER	BEFORE	AFTER
BLOOD SUGAR								
BLOOD PRESSURE								

Date __/__/__ Sunday	BREAKFAST		LUNCH		DINNER		BEDTIME	
	BEFORE	AFTER	BEFORE	AFTER	BEFORE	AFTER	BEFORE	AFTER
BLOOD SUGAR								
BLOOD PRESSURE								

NOTES: _____
_____
_____
_____

Month: _____ **Week Commencing:** _____

Date __/__/__	BREAKFAST		LUNCH		DINNER		BEDTIME	
Monday	BEFORE	AFTER	BEFORE	AFTER	BEFORE	AFTER	BEFORE	AFTER
BLOOD SUGAR								
BLOOD PRESSURE								
Date __/__/__	BREAKFAST		LUNCH		DINNER		BEDTIME	
Tuesday	BEFORE	AFTER	BEFORE	AFTER	BEFORE	AFTER	BEFORE	AFTER
BLOOD SUGAR								
BLOOD PRESSURE								
Date __/__/__	BREAKFAST		LUNCH		DINNER		BEDTIME	
Wednesday	BEFORE	AFTER	BEFORE	AFTER	BEFORE	AFTER	BEFORE	AFTER
BLOOD SUGAR								
BLOOD PRESSURE								
Date __/__/__	BREAKFAST		LUNCH		DINNER		BEDTIME	
Thursday	BEFORE	AFTER	BEFORE	AFTER	BEFORE	AFTER	BEFORE	AFTER
BLOOD SUGAR								
BLOOD PRESSURE								
Date __/__/__	BREAKFAST		LUNCH		DINNER		BEDTIME	
Friday	BEFORE	AFTER	BEFORE	AFTER	BEFORE	AFTER	BEFORE	AFTER
BLOOD SUGAR								
BLOOD PRESSURE								
Date __/__/__	BREAKFAST		LUNCH		DINNER		BEDTIME	
Saturday	BEFORE	AFTER	BEFORE	AFTER	BEFORE	AFTER	BEFORE	AFTER
BLOOD SUGAR								
BLOOD PRESSURE								
Date __/__/__	BREAKFAST		LUNCH		DINNER		BEDTIME	
Sunday	BEFORE	AFTER	BEFORE	AFTER	BEFORE	AFTER	BEFORE	AFTER
BLOOD SUGAR								
BLOOD PRESSURE								

NOTES: _____

_____

_____

Month: _____ **Week Commencing:** _____

Date __/__/__	BREAKFAST		LUNCH		DINNER		BEDTIME	
Monday	BEFORE	AFTER	BEFORE	AFTER	BEFORE	AFTER	BEFORE	AFTER
BLOOD SUGAR								
BLOOD PRESSURE								
Date __/__/__	BREAKFAST		LUNCH		DINNER		BEDTIME	
Tuesday	BEFORE	AFTER	BEFORE	AFTER	BEFORE	AFTER	BEFORE	AFTER
BLOOD SUGAR								
BLOOD PRESSURE								
Date __/__/__	BREAKFAST		LUNCH		DINNER		BEDTIME	
Wednesday	BEFORE	AFTER	BEFORE	AFTER	BEFORE	AFTER	BEFORE	AFTER
BLOOD SUGAR								
BLOOD PRESSURE								
Date __/__/__	BREAKFAST		LUNCH		DINNER		BEDTIME	
Thursday	BEFORE	AFTER	BEFORE	AFTER	BEFORE	AFTER	BEFORE	AFTER
BLOOD SUGAR								
BLOOD PRESSURE								
Date __/__/__	BREAKFAST		LUNCH		DINNER		BEDTIME	
Friday	BEFORE	AFTER	BEFORE	AFTER	BEFORE	AFTER	BEFORE	AFTER
BLOOD SUGAR								
BLOOD PRESSURE								
Date __/__/__	BREAKFAST		LUNCH		DINNER		BEDTIME	
Saturday	BEFORE	AFTER	BEFORE	AFTER	BEFORE	AFTER	BEFORE	AFTER
BLOOD SUGAR								
BLOOD PRESSURE								
Date __/__/__	BREAKFAST		LUNCH		DINNER		BEDTIME	
Sunday	BEFORE	AFTER	BEFORE	AFTER	BEFORE	AFTER	BEFORE	AFTER
BLOOD SUGAR								
BLOOD PRESSURE								

NOTES: _____

_____

_____

_____

Month: _____ **Week Commencing:** _____

Date __/__/__	BREAKFAST		LUNCH		DINNER		BEDTIME	
Monday	BEFORE	AFTER	BEFORE	AFTER	BEFORE	AFTER	BEFORE	AFTER
BLOOD SUGAR								
BLOOD PRESSURE								
Date __/__/__	BREAKFAST		LUNCH		DINNER		BEDTIME	
Tuesday	BEFORE	AFTER	BEFORE	AFTER	BEFORE	AFTER	BEFORE	AFTER
BLOOD SUGAR								
BLOOD PRESSURE								
Date __/__/__	BREAKFAST		LUNCH		DINNER		BEDTIME	
Wednesday	BEFORE	AFTER	BEFORE	AFTER	BEFORE	AFTER	BEFORE	AFTER
BLOOD SUGAR								
BLOOD PRESSURE								
Date __/__/__	BREAKFAST		LUNCH		DINNER		BEDTIME	
Thursday	BEFORE	AFTER	BEFORE	AFTER	BEFORE	AFTER	BEFORE	AFTER
BLOOD SUGAR								
BLOOD PRESSURE								
Date __/__/__	BREAKFAST		LUNCH		DINNER		BEDTIME	
Friday	BEFORE	AFTER	BEFORE	AFTER	BEFORE	AFTER	BEFORE	AFTER
BLOOD SUGAR								
BLOOD PRESSURE								
Date __/__/__	BREAKFAST		LUNCH		DINNER		BEDTIME	
Saturday	BEFORE	AFTER	BEFORE	AFTER	BEFORE	AFTER	BEFORE	AFTER
BLOOD SUGAR								
BLOOD PRESSURE								
Date __/__/__	BREAKFAST		LUNCH		DINNER		BEDTIME	
Sunday	BEFORE	AFTER	BEFORE	AFTER	BEFORE	AFTER	BEFORE	AFTER
BLOOD SUGAR								
BLOOD PRESSURE								

NOTES: _____
_____
_____
_____

Month: _____ Week Commencing: _____

Date __/__/__	BREAKFAST		LUNCH		DINNER		BEDTIME	
Monday	BEFORE	AFTER	BEFORE	AFTER	BEFORE	AFTER	BEFORE	AFTER
BLOOD SUGAR								
BLOOD PRESSURE								
Date __/__/__	BREAKFAST		LUNCH		DINNER		BEDTIME	
Tuesday	BEFORE	AFTER	BEFORE	AFTER	BEFORE	AFTER	BEFORE	AFTER
BLOOD SUGAR								
BLOOD PRESSURE								
Date __/__/__	BREAKFAST		LUNCH		DINNER		BEDTIME	
Wednesday	BEFORE	AFTER	BEFORE	AFTER	BEFORE	AFTER	BEFORE	AFTER
BLOOD SUGAR								
BLOOD PRESSURE								
Date __/__/__	BREAKFAST		LUNCH		DINNER		BEDTIME	
Thursday	BEFORE	AFTER	BEFORE	AFTER	BEFORE	AFTER	BEFORE	AFTER
BLOOD SUGAR								
BLOOD PRESSURE								
Date __/__/__	BREAKFAST		LUNCH		DINNER		BEDTIME	
Friday	BEFORE	AFTER	BEFORE	AFTER	BEFORE	AFTER	BEFORE	AFTER
BLOOD SUGAR								
BLOOD PRESSURE								
Date __/__/__	BREAKFAST		LUNCH		DINNER		BEDTIME	
Saturday	BEFORE	AFTER	BEFORE	AFTER	BEFORE	AFTER	BEFORE	AFTER
BLOOD SUGAR								
BLOOD PRESSURE								
Date __/__/__	BREAKFAST		LUNCH		DINNER		BEDTIME	
Sunday	BEFORE	AFTER	BEFORE	AFTER	BEFORE	AFTER	BEFORE	AFTER
BLOOD SUGAR								
BLOOD PRESSURE								

NOTES: _____
_____
_____
_____

Month: _____ **Week Commencing:** _____

Date __/__/__	BREAKFAST		LUNCH		DINNER		BEDTIME	
Monday	BEFORE	AFTER	BEFORE	AFTER	BEFORE	AFTER	BEFORE	AFTER
BLOOD SUGAR								
BLOOD PRESSURE								

Date __/__/__	BREAKFAST		LUNCH		DINNER		BEDTIME	
Tuesday	BEFORE	AFTER	BEFORE	AFTER	BEFORE	AFTER	BEFORE	AFTER
BLOOD SUGAR								
BLOOD PRESSURE								

Date __/__/__	BREAKFAST		LUNCH		DINNER		BEDTIME	
Wednesday	BEFORE	AFTER	BEFORE	AFTER	BEFORE	AFTER	BEFORE	AFTER
BLOOD SUGAR								
BLOOD PRESSURE								

Date __/__/__	BREAKFAST		LUNCH		DINNER		BEDTIME	
Thursday	BEFORE	AFTER	BEFORE	AFTER	BEFORE	AFTER	BEFORE	AFTER
BLOOD SUGAR								
BLOOD PRESSURE								

Date __/__/__	BREAKFAST		LUNCH		DINNER		BEDTIME	
Friday	BEFORE	AFTER	BEFORE	AFTER	BEFORE	AFTER	BEFORE	AFTER
BLOOD SUGAR								
BLOOD PRESSURE								

Date __/__/__	BREAKFAST		LUNCH		DINNER		BEDTIME	
Saturday	BEFORE	AFTER	BEFORE	AFTER	BEFORE	AFTER	BEFORE	AFTER
BLOOD SUGAR								
BLOOD PRESSURE								

Date __/__/__	BREAKFAST		LUNCH		DINNER		BEDTIME	
Sunday	BEFORE	AFTER	BEFORE	AFTER	BEFORE	AFTER	BEFORE	AFTER
BLOOD SUGAR								
BLOOD PRESSURE								

NOTES: _____
_____
_____
_____

Month: _____ **Week Commencing:** _____

Date __/__/__	BREAKFAST		LUNCH		DINNER		BEDTIME	
Monday	BEFORE	AFTER	BEFORE	AFTER	BEFORE	AFTER	BEFORE	AFTER
BLOOD SUGAR								
BLOOD PRESSURE								
Date __/__/__	BREAKFAST		LUNCH		DINNER		BEDTIME	
Tuesday	BEFORE	AFTER	BEFORE	AFTER	BEFORE	AFTER	BEFORE	AFTER
BLOOD SUGAR								
BLOOD PRESSURE								
Date __/__/__	BREAKFAST		LUNCH		DINNER		BEDTIME	
Wednesday	BEFORE	AFTER	BEFORE	AFTER	BEFORE	AFTER	BEFORE	AFTER
BLOOD SUGAR								
BLOOD PRESSURE								
Date __/__/__	BREAKFAST		LUNCH		DINNER		BEDTIME	
Thursday	BEFORE	AFTER	BEFORE	AFTER	BEFORE	AFTER	BEFORE	AFTER
BLOOD SUGAR								
BLOOD PRESSURE								
Date __/__/__	BREAKFAST		LUNCH		DINNER		BEDTIME	
Friday	BEFORE	AFTER	BEFORE	AFTER	BEFORE	AFTER	BEFORE	AFTER
BLOOD SUGAR								
BLOOD PRESSURE								
Date __/__/__	BREAKFAST		LUNCH		DINNER		BEDTIME	
Saturday	BEFORE	AFTER	BEFORE	AFTER	BEFORE	AFTER	BEFORE	AFTER
BLOOD SUGAR								
BLOOD PRESSURE								
Date __/__/__	BREAKFAST		LUNCH		DINNER		BEDTIME	
Sunday	BEFORE	AFTER	BEFORE	AFTER	BEFORE	AFTER	BEFORE	AFTER
BLOOD SUGAR								
BLOOD PRESSURE								

NOTES: _____
_____
_____
_____

Month: _____ **Week Commencing:** _____

Date __/__/__	BREAKFAST		LUNCH		DINNER		BEDTIME	
Monday	BEFORE	AFTER	BEFORE	AFTER	BEFORE	AFTER	BEFORE	AFTER
BLOOD SUGAR								
BLOOD PRESSURE								

Date __/__/__	BREAKFAST		LUNCH		DINNER		BEDTIME	
Tuesday	BEFORE	AFTER	BEFORE	AFTER	BEFORE	AFTER	BEFORE	AFTER
BLOOD SUGAR								
BLOOD PRESSURE								

Date __/__/__	BREAKFAST		LUNCH		DINNER		BEDTIME	
Wednesday	BEFORE	AFTER	BEFORE	AFTER	BEFORE	AFTER	BEFORE	AFTER
BLOOD SUGAR								
BLOOD PRESSURE								

Date __/__/__	BREAKFAST		LUNCH		DINNER		BEDTIME	
Thursday	BEFORE	AFTER	BEFORE	AFTER	BEFORE	AFTER	BEFORE	AFTER
BLOOD SUGAR								
BLOOD PRESSURE								

Date __/__/__	BREAKFAST		LUNCH		DINNER		BEDTIME	
Friday	BEFORE	AFTER	BEFORE	AFTER	BEFORE	AFTER	BEFORE	AFTER
BLOOD SUGAR								
BLOOD PRESSURE								

Date __/__/__	BREAKFAST		LUNCH		DINNER		BEDTIME	
Saturday	BEFORE	AFTER	BEFORE	AFTER	BEFORE	AFTER	BEFORE	AFTER
BLOOD SUGAR								
BLOOD PRESSURE								

Date __/__/__	BREAKFAST		LUNCH		DINNER		BEDTIME	
Sunday	BEFORE	AFTER	BEFORE	AFTER	BEFORE	AFTER	BEFORE	AFTER
BLOOD SUGAR								
BLOOD PRESSURE								

NOTES: _____
_____
_____
_____

Month: _____ **Week Commencing:** _____

Date __/__/__	BREAKFAST		LUNCH		DINNER		BEDTIME	
Monday	BEFORE	AFTER	BEFORE	AFTER	BEFORE	AFTER	BEFORE	AFTER
BLOOD SUGAR								
BLOOD PRESSURE								

Date __/__/__	BREAKFAST		LUNCH		DINNER		BEDTIME	
Tuesday	BEFORE	AFTER	BEFORE	AFTER	BEFORE	AFTER	BEFORE	AFTER
BLOOD SUGAR								
BLOOD PRESSURE								

Date __/__/__	BREAKFAST		LUNCH		DINNER		BEDTIME	
Wednesday	BEFORE	AFTER	BEFORE	AFTER	BEFORE	AFTER	BEFORE	AFTER
BLOOD SUGAR								
BLOOD PRESSURE								

Date __/__/__	BREAKFAST		LUNCH		DINNER		BEDTIME	
Thursday	BEFORE	AFTER	BEFORE	AFTER	BEFORE	AFTER	BEFORE	AFTER
BLOOD SUGAR								
BLOOD PRESSURE								

Date __/__/__	BREAKFAST		LUNCH		DINNER		BEDTIME	
Friday	BEFORE	AFTER	BEFORE	AFTER	BEFORE	AFTER	BEFORE	AFTER
BLOOD SUGAR								
BLOOD PRESSURE								

Date __/__/__	BREAKFAST		LUNCH		DINNER		BEDTIME	
Saturday	BEFORE	AFTER	BEFORE	AFTER	BEFORE	AFTER	BEFORE	AFTER
BLOOD SUGAR								
BLOOD PRESSURE								

Date __/__/__	BREAKFAST		LUNCH		DINNER		BEDTIME	
Sunday	BEFORE	AFTER	BEFORE	AFTER	BEFORE	AFTER	BEFORE	AFTER
BLOOD SUGAR								
BLOOD PRESSURE								

NOTES: _____
_____
_____
_____

Month: _____ **Week Commencing:** _____

Date ___/___/___	BREAKFAST		LUNCH		DINNER		BEDTIME	
Monday	BEFORE	AFTER	BEFORE	AFTER	BEFORE	AFTER	BEFORE	AFTER
BLOOD SUGAR								
BLOOD PRESSURE								
Date ___/___/___	BREAKFAST		LUNCH		DINNER		BEDTIME	
Tuesday	BEFORE	AFTER	BEFORE	AFTER	BEFORE	AFTER	BEFORE	AFTER
BLOOD SUGAR								
BLOOD PRESSURE								
Date ___/___/___	BREAKFAST		LUNCH		DINNER		BEDTIME	
Wednesday	BEFORE	AFTER	BEFORE	AFTER	BEFORE	AFTER	BEFORE	AFTER
BLOOD SUGAR								
BLOOD PRESSURE								
Date ___/___/___	BREAKFAST		LUNCH		DINNER		BEDTIME	
Thursday	BEFORE	AFTER	BEFORE	AFTER	BEFORE	AFTER	BEFORE	AFTER
BLOOD SUGAR								
BLOOD PRESSURE								
Date ___/___/___	BREAKFAST		LUNCH		DINNER		BEDTIME	
Friday	BEFORE	AFTER	BEFORE	AFTER	BEFORE	AFTER	BEFORE	AFTER
BLOOD SUGAR								
BLOOD PRESSURE								
Date ___/___/___	BREAKFAST		LUNCH		DINNER		BEDTIME	
Saturday	BEFORE	AFTER	BEFORE	AFTER	BEFORE	AFTER	BEFORE	AFTER
BLOOD SUGAR								
BLOOD PRESSURE								
Date ___/___/___	BREAKFAST		LUNCH		DINNER		BEDTIME	
Sunday	BEFORE	AFTER	BEFORE	AFTER	BEFORE	AFTER	BEFORE	AFTER
BLOOD SUGAR								
BLOOD PRESSURE								

NOTES: _____

_____

_____

_____

Month: _____ **Week Commencing:** _____

Date __/__/__	BREAKFAST		LUNCH		DINNER		BEDTIME	
Monday	BEFORE	AFTER	BEFORE	AFTER	BEFORE	AFTER	BEFORE	AFTER
BLOOD SUGAR								
BLOOD PRESSURE								
Date __/__/__	BREAKFAST		LUNCH		DINNER		BEDTIME	
Tuesday	BEFORE	AFTER	BEFORE	AFTER	BEFORE	AFTER	BEFORE	AFTER
BLOOD SUGAR								
BLOOD PRESSURE								
Date __/__/__	BREAKFAST		LUNCH		DINNER		BEDTIME	
Wednesday	BEFORE	AFTER	BEFORE	AFTER	BEFORE	AFTER	BEFORE	AFTER
BLOOD SUGAR								
BLOOD PRESSURE								
Date __/__/__	BREAKFAST		LUNCH		DINNER		BEDTIME	
Thursday	BEFORE	AFTER	BEFORE	AFTER	BEFORE	AFTER	BEFORE	AFTER
BLOOD SUGAR								
BLOOD PRESSURE								
Date __/__/__	BREAKFAST		LUNCH		DINNER		BEDTIME	
Friday	BEFORE	AFTER	BEFORE	AFTER	BEFORE	AFTER	BEFORE	AFTER
BLOOD SUGAR								
BLOOD PRESSURE								
Date __/__/__	BREAKFAST		LUNCH		DINNER		BEDTIME	
Saturday	BEFORE	AFTER	BEFORE	AFTER	BEFORE	AFTER	BEFORE	AFTER
BLOOD SUGAR								
BLOOD PRESSURE								
Date __/__/__	BREAKFAST		LUNCH		DINNER		BEDTIME	
Sunday	BEFORE	AFTER	BEFORE	AFTER	BEFORE	AFTER	BEFORE	AFTER
BLOOD SUGAR								
BLOOD PRESSURE								

NOTES: _____
_____
_____
_____

Month: _____ **Week Commencing:** _____

Date __/__/__	BREAKFAST		LUNCH		DINNER		BEDTIME	
Monday	BEFORE	AFTER	BEFORE	AFTER	BEFORE	AFTER	BEFORE	AFTER
BLOOD SUGAR								
BLOOD PRESSURE								
Date __/__/__	BREAKFAST		LUNCH		DINNER		BEDTIME	
Tuesday	BEFORE	AFTER	BEFORE	AFTER	BEFORE	AFTER	BEFORE	AFTER
BLOOD SUGAR								
BLOOD PRESSURE								
Date __/__/__	BREAKFAST		LUNCH		DINNER		BEDTIME	
Wednesday	BEFORE	AFTER	BEFORE	AFTER	BEFORE	AFTER	BEFORE	AFTER
BLOOD SUGAR								
BLOOD PRESSURE								
Date __/__/__	BREAKFAST		LUNCH		DINNER		BEDTIME	
Thursday	BEFORE	AFTER	BEFORE	AFTER	BEFORE	AFTER	BEFORE	AFTER
BLOOD SUGAR								
BLOOD PRESSURE								
Date __/__/__	BREAKFAST		LUNCH		DINNER		BEDTIME	
Friday	BEFORE	AFTER	BEFORE	AFTER	BEFORE	AFTER	BEFORE	AFTER
BLOOD SUGAR								
BLOOD PRESSURE								
Date __/__/__	BREAKFAST		LUNCH		DINNER		BEDTIME	
Saturday	BEFORE	AFTER	BEFORE	AFTER	BEFORE	AFTER	BEFORE	AFTER
BLOOD SUGAR								
BLOOD PRESSURE								
Date __/__/__	BREAKFAST		LUNCH		DINNER		BEDTIME	
Sunday	BEFORE	AFTER	BEFORE	AFTER	BEFORE	AFTER	BEFORE	AFTER
BLOOD SUGAR								
BLOOD PRESSURE								

NOTES: _____
_____
_____
_____

Month: _____ **Week Commencing:** _____

Date __/__/__	BREAKFAST		LUNCH		DINNER		BEDTIME	
Monday	BEFORE	AFTER	BEFORE	AFTER	BEFORE	AFTER	BEFORE	AFTER
BLOOD SUGAR								
BLOOD PRESSURE								
Date __/__/__	BREAKFAST		LUNCH		DINNER		BEDTIME	
Tuesday	BEFORE	AFTER	BEFORE	AFTER	BEFORE	AFTER	BEFORE	AFTER
BLOOD SUGAR								
BLOOD PRESSURE								
Date __/__/__	BREAKFAST		LUNCH		DINNER		BEDTIME	
Wednesday	BEFORE	AFTER	BEFORE	AFTER	BEFORE	AFTER	BEFORE	AFTER
BLOOD SUGAR								
BLOOD PRESSURE								
Date __/__/__	BREAKFAST		LUNCH		DINNER		BEDTIME	
Thursday	BEFORE	AFTER	BEFORE	AFTER	BEFORE	AFTER	BEFORE	AFTER
BLOOD SUGAR								
BLOOD PRESSURE								
Date __/__/__	BREAKFAST		LUNCH		DINNER		BEDTIME	
Friday	BEFORE	AFTER	BEFORE	AFTER	BEFORE	AFTER	BEFORE	AFTER
BLOOD SUGAR								
BLOOD PRESSURE								
Date __/__/__	BREAKFAST		LUNCH		DINNER		BEDTIME	
Saturday	BEFORE	AFTER	BEFORE	AFTER	BEFORE	AFTER	BEFORE	AFTER
BLOOD SUGAR								
BLOOD PRESSURE								
Date __/__/__	BREAKFAST		LUNCH		DINNER		BEDTIME	
Sunday	BEFORE	AFTER	BEFORE	AFTER	BEFORE	AFTER	BEFORE	AFTER
BLOOD SUGAR								
BLOOD PRESSURE								

NOTES: _____
_____
_____
_____

Month: _____   **Week Commencing:** _____

Date __/__/__	BREAKFAST		LUNCH		DINNER		BEDTIME	
Monday	BEFORE	AFTER	BEFORE	AFTER	BEFORE	AFTER	BEFORE	AFTER
BLOOD SUGAR								
BLOOD PRESSURE								
Date __/__/__	BREAKFAST		LUNCH		DINNER		BEDTIME	
Tuesday	BEFORE	AFTER	BEFORE	AFTER	BEFORE	AFTER	BEFORE	AFTER
BLOOD SUGAR								
BLOOD PRESSURE								
Date __/__/__	BREAKFAST		LUNCH		DINNER		BEDTIME	
Wednesday	BEFORE	AFTER	BEFORE	AFTER	BEFORE	AFTER	BEFORE	AFTER
BLOOD SUGAR								
BLOOD PRESSURE								
Date __/__/__	BREAKFAST		LUNCH		DINNER		BEDTIME	
Thursday	BEFORE	AFTER	BEFORE	AFTER	BEFORE	AFTER	BEFORE	AFTER
BLOOD SUGAR								
BLOOD PRESSURE								
Date __/__/__	BREAKFAST		LUNCH		DINNER		BEDTIME	
Friday	BEFORE	AFTER	BEFORE	AFTER	BEFORE	AFTER	BEFORE	AFTER
BLOOD SUGAR								
BLOOD PRESSURE								
Date __/__/__	BREAKFAST		LUNCH		DINNER		BEDTIME	
Saturday	BEFORE	AFTER	BEFORE	AFTER	BEFORE	AFTER	BEFORE	AFTER
BLOOD SUGAR								
BLOOD PRESSURE								
Date __/__/__	BREAKFAST		LUNCH		DINNER		BEDTIME	
Sunday	BEFORE	AFTER	BEFORE	AFTER	BEFORE	AFTER	BEFORE	AFTER
BLOOD SUGAR								
BLOOD PRESSURE								

NOTES: _____

_____

_____

Month: _____ **Week Commencing:** _____

Date __/__/__	BREAKFAST		LUNCH		DINNER		BEDTIME	
Monday	BEFORE	AFTER	BEFORE	AFTER	BEFORE	AFTER	BEFORE	AFTER
BLOOD SUGAR								
BLOOD PRESSURE								
Date __/__/__	BREAKFAST		LUNCH		DINNER		BEDTIME	
Tuesday	BEFORE	AFTER	BEFORE	AFTER	BEFORE	AFTER	BEFORE	AFTER
BLOOD SUGAR								
BLOOD PRESSURE								
Date __/__/__	BREAKFAST		LUNCH		DINNER		BEDTIME	
Wednesday	BEFORE	AFTER	BEFORE	AFTER	BEFORE	AFTER	BEFORE	AFTER
BLOOD SUGAR								
BLOOD PRESSURE								
Date __/__/__	BREAKFAST		LUNCH		DINNER		BEDTIME	
Thursday	BEFORE	AFTER	BEFORE	AFTER	BEFORE	AFTER	BEFORE	AFTER
BLOOD SUGAR								
BLOOD PRESSURE								
Date __/__/__	BREAKFAST		LUNCH		DINNER		BEDTIME	
Friday	BEFORE	AFTER	BEFORE	AFTER	BEFORE	AFTER	BEFORE	AFTER
BLOOD SUGAR								
BLOOD PRESSURE								
Date __/__/__	BREAKFAST		LUNCH		DINNER		BEDTIME	
Saturday	BEFORE	AFTER	BEFORE	AFTER	BEFORE	AFTER	BEFORE	AFTER
BLOOD SUGAR								
BLOOD PRESSURE								
Date __/__/__	BREAKFAST		LUNCH		DINNER		BEDTIME	
Sunday	BEFORE	AFTER	BEFORE	AFTER	BEFORE	AFTER	BEFORE	AFTER
BLOOD SUGAR								
BLOOD PRESSURE								

NOTES: _____
_____
_____
_____

Month: _____ **Week Commencing:** _____

Date __/__/__	BREAKFAST		LUNCH		DINNER		BEDTIME	
Monday	BEFORE	AFTER	BEFORE	AFTER	BEFORE	AFTER	BEFORE	AFTER
BLOOD SUGAR								
BLOOD PRESSURE								
Date __/__/__	BREAKFAST		LUNCH		DINNER		BEDTIME	
Tuesday	BEFORE	AFTER	BEFORE	AFTER	BEFORE	AFTER	BEFORE	AFTER
BLOOD SUGAR								
BLOOD PRESSURE								
Date __/__/__	BREAKFAST		LUNCH		DINNER		BEDTIME	
Wednesday	BEFORE	AFTER	BEFORE	AFTER	BEFORE	AFTER	BEFORE	AFTER
BLOOD SUGAR								
BLOOD PRESSURE								
Date __/__/__	BREAKFAST		LUNCH		DINNER		BEDTIME	
Thursday	BEFORE	AFTER	BEFORE	AFTER	BEFORE	AFTER	BEFORE	AFTER
BLOOD SUGAR								
BLOOD PRESSURE								
Date __/__/__	BREAKFAST		LUNCH		DINNER		BEDTIME	
Friday	BEFORE	AFTER	BEFORE	AFTER	BEFORE	AFTER	BEFORE	AFTER
BLOOD SUGAR								
BLOOD PRESSURE								
Date __/__/__	BREAKFAST		LUNCH		DINNER		BEDTIME	
Saturday	BEFORE	AFTER	BEFORE	AFTER	BEFORE	AFTER	BEFORE	AFTER
BLOOD SUGAR								
BLOOD PRESSURE								
Date __/__/__	BREAKFAST		LUNCH		DINNER		BEDTIME	
Sunday	BEFORE	AFTER	BEFORE	AFTER	BEFORE	AFTER	BEFORE	AFTER
BLOOD SUGAR								
BLOOD PRESSURE								

NOTES: _____

_____

_____

Month: _____ **Week Commencing:** _____

Date __/__/__	BREAKFAST		LUNCH		DINNER		BEDTIME	
Monday	BEFORE	AFTER	BEFORE	AFTER	BEFORE	AFTER	BEFORE	AFTER
BLOOD SUGAR								
BLOOD PRESSURE								
Date __/__/__	BREAKFAST		LUNCH		DINNER		BEDTIME	
Tuesday	BEFORE	AFTER	BEFORE	AFTER	BEFORE	AFTER	BEFORE	AFTER
BLOOD SUGAR								
BLOOD PRESSURE								
Date __/__/__	BREAKFAST		LUNCH		DINNER		BEDTIME	
Wednesday	BEFORE	AFTER	BEFORE	AFTER	BEFORE	AFTER	BEFORE	AFTER
BLOOD SUGAR								
BLOOD PRESSURE								
Date __/__/__	BREAKFAST		LUNCH		DINNER		BEDTIME	
Thursday	BEFORE	AFTER	BEFORE	AFTER	BEFORE	AFTER	BEFORE	AFTER
BLOOD SUGAR								
BLOOD PRESSURE								
Date __/__/__	BREAKFAST		LUNCH		DINNER		BEDTIME	
Friday	BEFORE	AFTER	BEFORE	AFTER	BEFORE	AFTER	BEFORE	AFTER
BLOOD SUGAR								
BLOOD PRESSURE								
Date __/__/__	BREAKFAST		LUNCH		DINNER		BEDTIME	
Saturday	BEFORE	AFTER	BEFORE	AFTER	BEFORE	AFTER	BEFORE	AFTER
BLOOD SUGAR								
BLOOD PRESSURE								
Date __/__/__	BREAKFAST		LUNCH		DINNER		BEDTIME	
Sunday	BEFORE	AFTER	BEFORE	AFTER	BEFORE	AFTER	BEFORE	AFTER
BLOOD SUGAR								
BLOOD PRESSURE								

NOTES: _____
_____
_____
_____

Month:									Week Commencing:	

Date __/__/__		BREAKFAST		LUNCH		DINNER		BEDTIME	
Monday		BEFORE	AFTER	BEFORE	AFTER	BEFORE	AFTER	BEFORE	AFTER
BLOOD SUGAR									
BLOOD PRESSURE									
Date __/__/__		BREAKFAST		LUNCH		DINNER		BEDTIME	
Tuesday		BEFORE	AFTER	BEFORE	AFTER	BEFORE	AFTER	BEFORE	AFTER
BLOOD SUGAR									
BLOOD PRESSURE									
Date __/__/__		BREAKFAST		LUNCH		DINNER		BEDTIME	
Wednesday		BEFORE	AFTER	BEFORE	AFTER	BEFORE	AFTER	BEFORE	AFTER
BLOOD SUGAR									
BLOOD PRESSURE									
Date __/__/__		BREAKFAST		LUNCH		DINNER		BEDTIME	
Thursday		BEFORE	AFTER	BEFORE	AFTER	BEFORE	AFTER	BEFORE	AFTER
BLOOD SUGAR									
BLOOD PRESSURE									
Date __/__/__		BREAKFAST		LUNCH		DINNER		BEDTIME	
Friday		BEFORE	AFTER	BEFORE	AFTER	BEFORE	AFTER	BEFORE	AFTER
BLOOD SUGAR									
BLOOD PRESSURE									
Date __/__/__		BREAKFAST		LUNCH		DINNER		BEDTIME	
Saturday		BEFORE	AFTER	BEFORE	AFTER	BEFORE	AFTER	BEFORE	AFTER
BLOOD SUGAR									
BLOOD PRESSURE									
Date __/__/__		BREAKFAST		LUNCH		DINNER		BEDTIME	
Sunday		BEFORE	AFTER	BEFORE	AFTER	BEFORE	AFTER	BEFORE	AFTER
BLOOD SUGAR									
BLOOD PRESSURE									

NOTES: _____

_____

_____

Month: _____ **Week Commencing:** _____

Date __/__/__	BREAKFAST		LUNCH		DINNER		BEDTIME	
Monday	BEFORE	AFTER	BEFORE	AFTER	BEFORE	AFTER	BEFORE	AFTER
BLOOD SUGAR								
BLOOD PRESSURE								
Date __/__/__	BREAKFAST		LUNCH		DINNER		BEDTIME	
Tuesday	BEFORE	AFTER	BEFORE	AFTER	BEFORE	AFTER	BEFORE	AFTER
BLOOD SUGAR								
BLOOD PRESSURE								
Date __/__/__	BREAKFAST		LUNCH		DINNER		BEDTIME	
Wednesday	BEFORE	AFTER	BEFORE	AFTER	BEFORE	AFTER	BEFORE	AFTER
BLOOD SUGAR								
BLOOD PRESSURE								
Date __/__/__	BREAKFAST		LUNCH		DINNER		BEDTIME	
Thursday	BEFORE	AFTER	BEFORE	AFTER	BEFORE	AFTER	BEFORE	AFTER
BLOOD SUGAR								
BLOOD PRESSURE								
Date __/__/__	BREAKFAST		LUNCH		DINNER		BEDTIME	
Friday	BEFORE	AFTER	BEFORE	AFTER	BEFORE	AFTER	BEFORE	AFTER
BLOOD SUGAR								
BLOOD PRESSURE								
Date __/__/__	BREAKFAST		LUNCH		DINNER		BEDTIME	
Saturday	BEFORE	AFTER	BEFORE	AFTER	BEFORE	AFTER	BEFORE	AFTER
BLOOD SUGAR								
BLOOD PRESSURE								
Date __/__/__	BREAKFAST		LUNCH		DINNER		BEDTIME	
Sunday	BEFORE	AFTER	BEFORE	AFTER	BEFORE	AFTER	BEFORE	AFTER
BLOOD SUGAR								
BLOOD PRESSURE								

NOTES: _____
_____
_____
_____

Month: _____ **Week Commencing:** _____

Date __/__/__	BREAKFAST		LUNCH		DINNER		BEDTIME	
Monday	BEFORE	AFTER	BEFORE	AFTER	BEFORE	AFTER	BEFORE	AFTER
BLOOD SUGAR								
BLOOD PRESSURE								
Date __/__/__	BREAKFAST		LUNCH		DINNER		BEDTIME	
Tuesday	BEFORE	AFTER	BEFORE	AFTER	BEFORE	AFTER	BEFORE	AFTER
BLOOD SUGAR								
BLOOD PRESSURE								
Date __/__/__	BREAKFAST		LUNCH		DINNER		BEDTIME	
Wednesday	BEFORE	AFTER	BEFORE	AFTER	BEFORE	AFTER	BEFORE	AFTER
BLOOD SUGAR								
BLOOD PRESSURE								
Date __/__/__	BREAKFAST		LUNCH		DINNER		BEDTIME	
Thursday	BEFORE	AFTER	BEFORE	AFTER	BEFORE	AFTER	BEFORE	AFTER
BLOOD SUGAR								
BLOOD PRESSURE								
Date __/__/__	BREAKFAST		LUNCH		DINNER		BEDTIME	
Friday	BEFORE	AFTER	BEFORE	AFTER	BEFORE	AFTER	BEFORE	AFTER
BLOOD SUGAR								
BLOOD PRESSURE								
Date __/__/__	BREAKFAST		LUNCH		DINNER		BEDTIME	
Saturday	BEFORE	AFTER	BEFORE	AFTER	BEFORE	AFTER	BEFORE	AFTER
BLOOD SUGAR								
BLOOD PRESSURE								
Date __/__/__	BREAKFAST		LUNCH		DINNER		BEDTIME	
Sunday	BEFORE	AFTER	BEFORE	AFTER	BEFORE	AFTER	BEFORE	AFTER
BLOOD SUGAR								
BLOOD PRESSURE								

NOTES: _____

_____

_____

Month: _____ **Week Commencing:** _____

Date __/__/__	BREAKFAST		LUNCH		DINNER		BEDTIME	
Monday	BEFORE	AFTER	BEFORE	AFTER	BEFORE	AFTER	BEFORE	AFTER
BLOOD SUGAR								
BLOOD PRESSURE								
Date __/__/__	BREAKFAST		LUNCH		DINNER		BEDTIME	
Tuesday	BEFORE	AFTER	BEFORE	AFTER	BEFORE	AFTER	BEFORE	AFTER
BLOOD SUGAR								
BLOOD PRESSURE								
Date __/__/__	BREAKFAST		LUNCH		DINNER		BEDTIME	
Wednesday	BEFORE	AFTER	BEFORE	AFTER	BEFORE	AFTER	BEFORE	AFTER
BLOOD SUGAR								
BLOOD PRESSURE								
Date __/__/__	BREAKFAST		LUNCH		DINNER		BEDTIME	
Thursday	BEFORE	AFTER	BEFORE	AFTER	BEFORE	AFTER	BEFORE	AFTER
BLOOD SUGAR								
BLOOD PRESSURE								
Date __/__/__	BREAKFAST		LUNCH		DINNER		BEDTIME	
Friday	BEFORE	AFTER	BEFORE	AFTER	BEFORE	AFTER	BEFORE	AFTER
BLOOD SUGAR								
BLOOD PRESSURE								
Date __/__/__	BREAKFAST		LUNCH		DINNER		BEDTIME	
Saturday	BEFORE	AFTER	BEFORE	AFTER	BEFORE	AFTER	BEFORE	AFTER
BLOOD SUGAR								
BLOOD PRESSURE								
Date __/__/__	BREAKFAST		LUNCH		DINNER		BEDTIME	
Sunday	BEFORE	AFTER	BEFORE	AFTER	BEFORE	AFTER	BEFORE	AFTER
BLOOD SUGAR								
BLOOD PRESSURE								

NOTES: _____
_____
_____
_____

Month: _____ **Week Commencing:** _____

Date __/__/__	BREAKFAST		LUNCH		DINNER		BEDTIME	
Monday	BEFORE	AFTER	BEFORE	AFTER	BEFORE	AFTER	BEFORE	AFTER
BLOOD SUGAR								
BLOOD PRESSURE								
Date __/__/__	BREAKFAST		LUNCH		DINNER		BEDTIME	
Tuesday	BEFORE	AFTER	BEFORE	AFTER	BEFORE	AFTER	BEFORE	AFTER
BLOOD SUGAR								
BLOOD PRESSURE								
Date __/__/__	BREAKFAST		LUNCH		DINNER		BEDTIME	
Wednesday	BEFORE	AFTER	BEFORE	AFTER	BEFORE	AFTER	BEFORE	AFTER
BLOOD SUGAR								
BLOOD PRESSURE								
Date __/__/__	BREAKFAST		LUNCH		DINNER		BEDTIME	
Thursday	BEFORE	AFTER	BEFORE	AFTER	BEFORE	AFTER	BEFORE	AFTER
BLOOD SUGAR								
BLOOD PRESSURE								
Date __/__/__	BREAKFAST		LUNCH		DINNER		BEDTIME	
Friday	BEFORE	AFTER	BEFORE	AFTER	BEFORE	AFTER	BEFORE	AFTER
BLOOD SUGAR								
BLOOD PRESSURE								
Date __/__/__	BREAKFAST		LUNCH		DINNER		BEDTIME	
Saturday	BEFORE	AFTER	BEFORE	AFTER	BEFORE	AFTER	BEFORE	AFTER
BLOOD SUGAR								
BLOOD PRESSURE								
Date __/__/__	BREAKFAST		LUNCH		DINNER		BEDTIME	
Sunday	BEFORE	AFTER	BEFORE	AFTER	BEFORE	AFTER	BEFORE	AFTER
BLOOD SUGAR								
BLOOD PRESSURE								

NOTES: _____

_____

_____

Month: _____ **Week Commencing:** _____

Date __/__/__	BREAKFAST		LUNCH		DINNER		BEDTIME	
Monday	BEFORE	AFTER	BEFORE	AFTER	BEFORE	AFTER	BEFORE	AFTER
BLOOD SUGAR								
BLOOD PRESSURE								
Date __/__/__	BREAKFAST		LUNCH		DINNER		BEDTIME	
Tuesday	BEFORE	AFTER	BEFORE	AFTER	BEFORE	AFTER	BEFORE	AFTER
BLOOD SUGAR								
BLOOD PRESSURE								
Date __/__/__	BREAKFAST		LUNCH		DINNER		BEDTIME	
Wednesday	BEFORE	AFTER	BEFORE	AFTER	BEFORE	AFTER	BEFORE	AFTER
BLOOD SUGAR								
BLOOD PRESSURE								
Date __/__/__	BREAKFAST		LUNCH		DINNER		BEDTIME	
Thursday	BEFORE	AFTER	BEFORE	AFTER	BEFORE	AFTER	BEFORE	AFTER
BLOOD SUGAR								
BLOOD PRESSURE								
Date __/__/__	BREAKFAST		LUNCH		DINNER		BEDTIME	
Friday	BEFORE	AFTER	BEFORE	AFTER	BEFORE	AFTER	BEFORE	AFTER
BLOOD SUGAR								
BLOOD PRESSURE								
Date __/__/__	BREAKFAST		LUNCH		DINNER		BEDTIME	
Saturday	BEFORE	AFTER	BEFORE	AFTER	BEFORE	AFTER	BEFORE	AFTER
BLOOD SUGAR								
BLOOD PRESSURE								
Date __/__/__	BREAKFAST		LUNCH		DINNER		BEDTIME	
Sunday	BEFORE	AFTER	BEFORE	AFTER	BEFORE	AFTER	BEFORE	AFTER
BLOOD SUGAR								
BLOOD PRESSURE								

NOTES: _____
_____
_____
_____

Month: _____ **Week Commencing:** _____

Date __/__/__	BREAKFAST		LUNCH		DINNER		BEDTIME	
Monday	BEFORE	AFTER	BEFORE	AFTER	BEFORE	AFTER	BEFORE	AFTER
BLOOD SUGAR								
BLOOD PRESSURE								
Date __/__/__	BREAKFAST		LUNCH		DINNER		BEDTIME	
Tuesday	BEFORE	AFTER	BEFORE	AFTER	BEFORE	AFTER	BEFORE	AFTER
BLOOD SUGAR								
BLOOD PRESSURE								
Date __/__/__	BREAKFAST		LUNCH		DINNER		BEDTIME	
Wednesday	BEFORE	AFTER	BEFORE	AFTER	BEFORE	AFTER	BEFORE	AFTER
BLOOD SUGAR								
BLOOD PRESSURE								
Date __/__/__	BREAKFAST		LUNCH		DINNER		BEDTIME	
Thursday	BEFORE	AFTER	BEFORE	AFTER	BEFORE	AFTER	BEFORE	AFTER
BLOOD SUGAR								
BLOOD PRESSURE								
Date __/__/__	BREAKFAST		LUNCH		DINNER		BEDTIME	
Friday	BEFORE	AFTER	BEFORE	AFTER	BEFORE	AFTER	BEFORE	AFTER
BLOOD SUGAR								
BLOOD PRESSURE								
Date __/__/__	BREAKFAST		LUNCH		DINNER		BEDTIME	
Saturday	BEFORE	AFTER	BEFORE	AFTER	BEFORE	AFTER	BEFORE	AFTER
BLOOD SUGAR								
BLOOD PRESSURE								
Date __/__/__	BREAKFAST		LUNCH		DINNER		BEDTIME	
Sunday	BEFORE	AFTER	BEFORE	AFTER	BEFORE	AFTER	BEFORE	AFTER
BLOOD SUGAR								
BLOOD PRESSURE								

NOTES: _____
_____
_____
_____

Month: _____ **Week Commencing:** _____

Date __/__/__	BREAKFAST		LUNCH		DINNER		BEDTIME	
Monday	BEFORE	AFTER	BEFORE	AFTER	BEFORE	AFTER	BEFORE	AFTER
BLOOD SUGAR								
BLOOD PRESSURE								
Date __/__/__	BREAKFAST		LUNCH		DINNER		BEDTIME	
Tuesday	BEFORE	AFTER	BEFORE	AFTER	BEFORE	AFTER	BEFORE	AFTER
BLOOD SUGAR								
BLOOD PRESSURE								
Date __/__/__	BREAKFAST		LUNCH		DINNER		BEDTIME	
Wednesday	BEFORE	AFTER	BEFORE	AFTER	BEFORE	AFTER	BEFORE	AFTER
BLOOD SUGAR								
BLOOD PRESSURE								
Date __/__/__	BREAKFAST		LUNCH		DINNER		BEDTIME	
Thursday	BEFORE	AFTER	BEFORE	AFTER	BEFORE	AFTER	BEFORE	AFTER
BLOOD SUGAR								
BLOOD PRESSURE								
Date __/__/__	BREAKFAST		LUNCH		DINNER		BEDTIME	
Friday	BEFORE	AFTER	BEFORE	AFTER	BEFORE	AFTER	BEFORE	AFTER
BLOOD SUGAR								
BLOOD PRESSURE								
Date __/__/__	BREAKFAST		LUNCH		DINNER		BEDTIME	
Saturday	BEFORE	AFTER	BEFORE	AFTER	BEFORE	AFTER	BEFORE	AFTER
BLOOD SUGAR								
BLOOD PRESSURE								
Date __/__/__	BREAKFAST		LUNCH		DINNER		BEDTIME	
Sunday	BEFORE	AFTER	BEFORE	AFTER	BEFORE	AFTER	BEFORE	AFTER
BLOOD SUGAR								
BLOOD PRESSURE								

NOTES: _____
_____
_____
_____

Month: _____ **Week Commencing:** _____

Date __/__/__	BREAKFAST		LUNCH		DINNER		BEDTIME	
Monday	BEFORE	AFTER	BEFORE	AFTER	BEFORE	AFTER	BEFORE	AFTER
BLOOD SUGAR								
BLOOD PRESSURE								
Date __/__/__	BREAKFAST		LUNCH		DINNER		BEDTIME	
Tuesday	BEFORE	AFTER	BEFORE	AFTER	BEFORE	AFTER	BEFORE	AFTER
BLOOD SUGAR								
BLOOD PRESSURE								
Date __/__/__	BREAKFAST		LUNCH		DINNER		BEDTIME	
Wednesday	BEFORE	AFTER	BEFORE	AFTER	BEFORE	AFTER	BEFORE	AFTER
BLOOD SUGAR								
BLOOD PRESSURE								
Date __/__/__	BREAKFAST		LUNCH		DINNER		BEDTIME	
Thursday	BEFORE	AFTER	BEFORE	AFTER	BEFORE	AFTER	BEFORE	AFTER
BLOOD SUGAR								
BLOOD PRESSURE								
Date __/__/__	BREAKFAST		LUNCH		DINNER		BEDTIME	
Friday	BEFORE	AFTER	BEFORE	AFTER	BEFORE	AFTER	BEFORE	AFTER
BLOOD SUGAR								
BLOOD PRESSURE								
Date __/__/__	BREAKFAST		LUNCH		DINNER		BEDTIME	
Saturday	BEFORE	AFTER	BEFORE	AFTER	BEFORE	AFTER	BEFORE	AFTER
BLOOD SUGAR								
BLOOD PRESSURE								
Date __/__/__	BREAKFAST		LUNCH		DINNER		BEDTIME	
Sunday	BEFORE	AFTER	BEFORE	AFTER	BEFORE	AFTER	BEFORE	AFTER
BLOOD SUGAR								
BLOOD PRESSURE								

NOTES: _____

_____

_____

Month: _____ **Week Commencing:** _____

Date __/__/__ Monday	BREAKFAST		LUNCH		DINNER		BEDTIME	
	BEFORE	AFTER	BEFORE	AFTER	BEFORE	AFTER	BEFORE	AFTER
BLOOD SUGAR								
BLOOD PRESSURE								

Date __/__/__ Tuesday	BREAKFAST		LUNCH		DINNER		BEDTIME	
	BEFORE	AFTER	BEFORE	AFTER	BEFORE	AFTER	BEFORE	AFTER
BLOOD SUGAR								
BLOOD PRESSURE								

Date __/__/__ Wednesday	BREAKFAST		LUNCH		DINNER		BEDTIME	
	BEFORE	AFTER	BEFORE	AFTER	BEFORE	AFTER	BEFORE	AFTER
BLOOD SUGAR								
BLOOD PRESSURE								

Date __/__/__ Thursday	BREAKFAST		LUNCH		DINNER		BEDTIME	
	BEFORE	AFTER	BEFORE	AFTER	BEFORE	AFTER	BEFORE	AFTER
BLOOD SUGAR								
BLOOD PRESSURE								

Date __/__/__ Friday	BREAKFAST		LUNCH		DINNER		BEDTIME	
	BEFORE	AFTER	BEFORE	AFTER	BEFORE	AFTER	BEFORE	AFTER
BLOOD SUGAR								
BLOOD PRESSURE								

Date __/__/__ Saturday	BREAKFAST		LUNCH		DINNER		BEDTIME	
	BEFORE	AFTER	BEFORE	AFTER	BEFORE	AFTER	BEFORE	AFTER
BLOOD SUGAR								
BLOOD PRESSURE								

Date __/__/__ Sunday	BREAKFAST		LUNCH		DINNER		BEDTIME	
	BEFORE	AFTER	BEFORE	AFTER	BEFORE	AFTER	BEFORE	AFTER
BLOOD SUGAR								
BLOOD PRESSURE								

NOTES: _____
_____
_____
_____

Month: _____ Week Commencing: _____

Date ___/___/___	BREAKFAST		LUNCH		DINNER		BEDTIME	
Monday	BEFORE	AFTER	BEFORE	AFTER	BEFORE	AFTER	BEFORE	AFTER
BLOOD SUGAR								
BLOOD PRESSURE								
Date ___/___/___	BREAKFAST		LUNCH		DINNER		BEDTIME	
Tuesday	BEFORE	AFTER	BEFORE	AFTER	BEFORE	AFTER	BEFORE	AFTER
BLOOD SUGAR								
BLOOD PRESSURE								
Date ___/___/___	BREAKFAST		LUNCH		DINNER		BEDTIME	
Wednesday	BEFORE	AFTER	BEFORE	AFTER	BEFORE	AFTER	BEFORE	AFTER
BLOOD SUGAR								
BLOOD PRESSURE								
Date ___/___/___	BREAKFAST		LUNCH		DINNER		BEDTIME	
Thursday	BEFORE	AFTER	BEFORE	AFTER	BEFORE	AFTER	BEFORE	AFTER
BLOOD SUGAR								
BLOOD PRESSURE								
Date ___/___/___	BREAKFAST		LUNCH		DINNER		BEDTIME	
Friday	BEFORE	AFTER	BEFORE	AFTER	BEFORE	AFTER	BEFORE	AFTER
BLOOD SUGAR								
BLOOD PRESSURE								
Date ___/___/___	BREAKFAST		LUNCH		DINNER		BEDTIME	
Saturday	BEFORE	AFTER	BEFORE	AFTER	BEFORE	AFTER	BEFORE	AFTER
BLOOD SUGAR								
BLOOD PRESSURE								
Date ___/___/___	BREAKFAST		LUNCH		DINNER		BEDTIME	
Sunday	BEFORE	AFTER	BEFORE	AFTER	BEFORE	AFTER	BEFORE	AFTER
BLOOD SUGAR								
BLOOD PRESSURE								

NOTES: _____
_____
_____

Month: _____ **Week Commencing:** _____

Date __/__/__	BREAKFAST		LUNCH		DINNER		BEDTIME	
Monday	BEFORE	AFTER	BEFORE	AFTER	BEFORE	AFTER	BEFORE	AFTER
BLOOD SUGAR								
BLOOD PRESSURE								
Date __/__/__	BREAKFAST		LUNCH		DINNER		BEDTIME	
Tuesday	BEFORE	AFTER	BEFORE	AFTER	BEFORE	AFTER	BEFORE	AFTER
BLOOD SUGAR								
BLOOD PRESSURE								
Date __/__/__	BREAKFAST		LUNCH		DINNER		BEDTIME	
Wednesday	BEFORE	AFTER	BEFORE	AFTER	BEFORE	AFTER	BEFORE	AFTER
BLOOD SUGAR								
BLOOD PRESSURE								
Date __/__/__	BREAKFAST		LUNCH		DINNER		BEDTIME	
Thursday	BEFORE	AFTER	BEFORE	AFTER	BEFORE	AFTER	BEFORE	AFTER
BLOOD SUGAR								
BLOOD PRESSURE								
Date __/__/__	BREAKFAST		LUNCH		DINNER		BEDTIME	
Friday	BEFORE	AFTER	BEFORE	AFTER	BEFORE	AFTER	BEFORE	AFTER
BLOOD SUGAR								
BLOOD PRESSURE								
Date __/__/__	BREAKFAST		LUNCH		DINNER		BEDTIME	
Saturday	BEFORE	AFTER	BEFORE	AFTER	BEFORE	AFTER	BEFORE	AFTER
BLOOD SUGAR								
BLOOD PRESSURE								
Date __/__/__	BREAKFAST		LUNCH		DINNER		BEDTIME	
Sunday	BEFORE	AFTER	BEFORE	AFTER	BEFORE	AFTER	BEFORE	AFTER
BLOOD SUGAR								
BLOOD PRESSURE								

NOTES: _____
_____
_____
_____

Month: _____ **Week Commencing:** _____

Date __/__/__	BREAKFAST		LUNCH		DINNER		BEDTIME	
Monday	BEFORE	AFTER	BEFORE	AFTER	BEFORE	AFTER	BEFORE	AFTER
BLOOD SUGAR								
BLOOD PRESSURE								
Date __/__/__	BREAKFAST		LUNCH		DINNER		BEDTIME	
Tuesday	BEFORE	AFTER	BEFORE	AFTER	BEFORE	AFTER	BEFORE	AFTER
BLOOD SUGAR								
BLOOD PRESSURE								
Date __/__/__	BREAKFAST		LUNCH		DINNER		BEDTIME	
Wednesday	BEFORE	AFTER	BEFORE	AFTER	BEFORE	AFTER	BEFORE	AFTER
BLOOD SUGAR								
BLOOD PRESSURE								
Date __/__/__	BREAKFAST		LUNCH		DINNER		BEDTIME	
Thursday	BEFORE	AFTER	BEFORE	AFTER	BEFORE	AFTER	BEFORE	AFTER
BLOOD SUGAR								
BLOOD PRESSURE								
Date __/__/__	BREAKFAST		LUNCH		DINNER		BEDTIME	
Friday	BEFORE	AFTER	BEFORE	AFTER	BEFORE	AFTER	BEFORE	AFTER
BLOOD SUGAR								
BLOOD PRESSURE								
Date __/__/__	BREAKFAST		LUNCH		DINNER		BEDTIME	
Saturday	BEFORE	AFTER	BEFORE	AFTER	BEFORE	AFTER	BEFORE	AFTER
BLOOD SUGAR								
BLOOD PRESSURE								
Date __/__/__	BREAKFAST		LUNCH		DINNER		BEDTIME	
Sunday	BEFORE	AFTER	BEFORE	AFTER	BEFORE	AFTER	BEFORE	AFTER
BLOOD SUGAR								
BLOOD PRESSURE								

NOTES: _____

_____

_____

_____

Month: _____ **Week Commencing:** _____

Date __/__/__	BREAKFAST		LUNCH		DINNER		BEDTIME	
Monday	BEFORE	AFTER	BEFORE	AFTER	BEFORE	AFTER	BEFORE	AFTER
BLOOD SUGAR								
BLOOD PRESSURE								
Date __/__/__	BREAKFAST		LUNCH		DINNER		BEDTIME	
Tuesday	BEFORE	AFTER	BEFORE	AFTER	BEFORE	AFTER	BEFORE	AFTER
BLOOD SUGAR								
BLOOD PRESSURE								
Date __/__/__	BREAKFAST		LUNCH		DINNER		BEDTIME	
Wednesday	BEFORE	AFTER	BEFORE	AFTER	BEFORE	AFTER	BEFORE	AFTER
BLOOD SUGAR								
BLOOD PRESSURE								
Date __/__/__	BREAKFAST		LUNCH		DINNER		BEDTIME	
Thursday	BEFORE	AFTER	BEFORE	AFTER	BEFORE	AFTER	BEFORE	AFTER
BLOOD SUGAR								
BLOOD PRESSURE								
Date __/__/__	BREAKFAST		LUNCH		DINNER		BEDTIME	
Friday	BEFORE	AFTER	BEFORE	AFTER	BEFORE	AFTER	BEFORE	AFTER
BLOOD SUGAR								
BLOOD PRESSURE								
Date __/__/__	BREAKFAST		LUNCH		DINNER		BEDTIME	
Saturday	BEFORE	AFTER	BEFORE	AFTER	BEFORE	AFTER	BEFORE	AFTER
BLOOD SUGAR								
BLOOD PRESSURE								
Date __/__/__	BREAKFAST		LUNCH		DINNER		BEDTIME	
Sunday	BEFORE	AFTER	BEFORE	AFTER	BEFORE	AFTER	BEFORE	AFTER
BLOOD SUGAR								
BLOOD PRESSURE								

NOTES: _____
_____
_____
_____

Month: _____ **Week Commencing:** _____

Date ___/___/___	BREAKFAST		LUNCH		DINNER		BEDTIME	
Monday	BEFORE	AFTER	BEFORE	AFTER	BEFORE	AFTER	BEFORE	AFTER
BLOOD SUGAR								
BLOOD PRESSURE								
Date ___/___/___	BREAKFAST		LUNCH		DINNER		BEDTIME	
Tuesday	BEFORE	AFTER	BEFORE	AFTER	BEFORE	AFTER	BEFORE	AFTER
BLOOD SUGAR								
BLOOD PRESSURE								
Date ___/___/___	BREAKFAST		LUNCH		DINNER		BEDTIME	
Wednesday	BEFORE	AFTER	BEFORE	AFTER	BEFORE	AFTER	BEFORE	AFTER
BLOOD SUGAR								
BLOOD PRESSURE								
Date ___/___/___	BREAKFAST		LUNCH		DINNER		BEDTIME	
Thursday	BEFORE	AFTER	BEFORE	AFTER	BEFORE	AFTER	BEFORE	AFTER
BLOOD SUGAR								
BLOOD PRESSURE								
Date ___/___/___	BREAKFAST		LUNCH		DINNER		BEDTIME	
Friday	BEFORE	AFTER	BEFORE	AFTER	BEFORE	AFTER	BEFORE	AFTER
BLOOD SUGAR								
BLOOD PRESSURE								
Date ___/___/___	BREAKFAST		LUNCH		DINNER		BEDTIME	
Saturday	BEFORE	AFTER	BEFORE	AFTER	BEFORE	AFTER	BEFORE	AFTER
BLOOD SUGAR								
BLOOD PRESSURE								
Date ___/___/___	BREAKFAST		LUNCH		DINNER		BEDTIME	
Sunday	BEFORE	AFTER	BEFORE	AFTER	BEFORE	AFTER	BEFORE	AFTER
BLOOD SUGAR								
BLOOD PRESSURE								

NOTES: _____

_____

_____

Month: _____ **Week Commencing:** _____

Date __/__/__	BREAKFAST		LUNCH		DINNER		BEDTIME	
Monday	BEFORE	AFTER	BEFORE	AFTER	BEFORE	AFTER	BEFORE	AFTER
BLOOD SUGAR								
BLOOD PRESSURE								
Date __/__/__	BREAKFAST		LUNCH		DINNER		BEDTIME	
Tuesday	BEFORE	AFTER	BEFORE	AFTER	BEFORE	AFTER	BEFORE	AFTER
BLOOD SUGAR								
BLOOD PRESSURE								
Date __/__/__	BREAKFAST		LUNCH		DINNER		BEDTIME	
Wednesday	BEFORE	AFTER	BEFORE	AFTER	BEFORE	AFTER	BEFORE	AFTER
BLOOD SUGAR								
BLOOD PRESSURE								
Date __/__/__	BREAKFAST		LUNCH		DINNER		BEDTIME	
Thursday	BEFORE	AFTER	BEFORE	AFTER	BEFORE	AFTER	BEFORE	AFTER
BLOOD SUGAR								
BLOOD PRESSURE								
Date __/__/__	BREAKFAST		LUNCH		DINNER		BEDTIME	
Friday	BEFORE	AFTER	BEFORE	AFTER	BEFORE	AFTER	BEFORE	AFTER
BLOOD SUGAR								
BLOOD PRESSURE								
Date __/__/__	BREAKFAST		LUNCH		DINNER		BEDTIME	
Saturday	BEFORE	AFTER	BEFORE	AFTER	BEFORE	AFTER	BEFORE	AFTER
BLOOD SUGAR								
BLOOD PRESSURE								
Date __/__/__	BREAKFAST		LUNCH		DINNER		BEDTIME	
Sunday	BEFORE	AFTER	BEFORE	AFTER	BEFORE	AFTER	BEFORE	AFTER
BLOOD SUGAR								
BLOOD PRESSURE								

NOTES: _____
_____
_____
_____

Month: _____ **Week Commencing:** _____

Date __/__/__	BREAKFAST		LUNCH		DINNER		BEDTIME	
Monday	BEFORE	AFTER	BEFORE	AFTER	BEFORE	AFTER	BEFORE	AFTER
BLOOD SUGAR								
BLOOD PRESSURE								
Date __/__/__	BREAKFAST		LUNCH		DINNER		BEDTIME	
Tuesday	BEFORE	AFTER	BEFORE	AFTER	BEFORE	AFTER	BEFORE	AFTER
BLOOD SUGAR								
BLOOD PRESSURE								
Date __/__/__	BREAKFAST		LUNCH		DINNER		BEDTIME	
Wednesday	BEFORE	AFTER	BEFORE	AFTER	BEFORE	AFTER	BEFORE	AFTER
BLOOD SUGAR								
BLOOD PRESSURE								
Date __/__/__	BREAKFAST		LUNCH		DINNER		BEDTIME	
Thursday	BEFORE	AFTER	BEFORE	AFTER	BEFORE	AFTER	BEFORE	AFTER
BLOOD SUGAR								
BLOOD PRESSURE								
Date __/__/__	BREAKFAST		LUNCH		DINNER		BEDTIME	
Friday	BEFORE	AFTER	BEFORE	AFTER	BEFORE	AFTER	BEFORE	AFTER
BLOOD SUGAR								
BLOOD PRESSURE								
Date __/__/__	BREAKFAST		LUNCH		DINNER		BEDTIME	
Saturday	BEFORE	AFTER	BEFORE	AFTER	BEFORE	AFTER	BEFORE	AFTER
BLOOD SUGAR								
BLOOD PRESSURE								
Date __/__/__	BREAKFAST		LUNCH		DINNER		BEDTIME	
Sunday	BEFORE	AFTER	BEFORE	AFTER	BEFORE	AFTER	BEFORE	AFTER
BLOOD SUGAR								
BLOOD PRESSURE								

NOTES: _____

_____

_____

Month: _____ **Week Commencing:** _____

Date __/__/__ Monday	BREAKFAST		LUNCH		DINNER		BEDTIME	
	BEFORE	AFTER	BEFORE	AFTER	BEFORE	AFTER	BEFORE	AFTER
BLOOD SUGAR								
BLOOD PRESSURE								

Date __/__/__ Tuesday	BREAKFAST		LUNCH		DINNER		BEDTIME	
	BEFORE	AFTER	BEFORE	AFTER	BEFORE	AFTER	BEFORE	AFTER
BLOOD SUGAR								
BLOOD PRESSURE								

Date __/__/__ Wednesday	BREAKFAST		LUNCH		DINNER		BEDTIME	
	BEFORE	AFTER	BEFORE	AFTER	BEFORE	AFTER	BEFORE	AFTER
BLOOD SUGAR								
BLOOD PRESSURE								

Date __/__/__ Thursday	BREAKFAST		LUNCH		DINNER		BEDTIME	
	BEFORE	AFTER	BEFORE	AFTER	BEFORE	AFTER	BEFORE	AFTER
BLOOD SUGAR								
BLOOD PRESSURE								

Date __/__/__ Friday	BREAKFAST		LUNCH		DINNER		BEDTIME	
	BEFORE	AFTER	BEFORE	AFTER	BEFORE	AFTER	BEFORE	AFTER
BLOOD SUGAR								
BLOOD PRESSURE								

Date __/__/__ Saturday	BREAKFAST		LUNCH		DINNER		BEDTIME	
	BEFORE	AFTER	BEFORE	AFTER	BEFORE	AFTER	BEFORE	AFTER
BLOOD SUGAR								
BLOOD PRESSURE								

Date __/__/__ Sunday	BREAKFAST		LUNCH		DINNER		BEDTIME	
	BEFORE	AFTER	BEFORE	AFTER	BEFORE	AFTER	BEFORE	AFTER
BLOOD SUGAR								
BLOOD PRESSURE								

NOTES: _____
_____
_____
_____

Month: _____ **Week Commencing:** _____

Date __/__/__	BREAKFAST		LUNCH		DINNER		BEDTIME	
Monday	BEFORE	AFTER	BEFORE	AFTER	BEFORE	AFTER	BEFORE	AFTER
BLOOD SUGAR								
BLOOD PRESSURE								
Date __/__/__	BREAKFAST		LUNCH		DINNER		BEDTIME	
Tuesday	BEFORE	AFTER	BEFORE	AFTER	BEFORE	AFTER	BEFORE	AFTER
BLOOD SUGAR								
BLOOD PRESSURE								
Date __/__/__	BREAKFAST		LUNCH		DINNER		BEDTIME	
Wednesday	BEFORE	AFTER	BEFORE	AFTER	BEFORE	AFTER	BEFORE	AFTER
BLOOD SUGAR								
BLOOD PRESSURE								
Date __/__/__	BREAKFAST		LUNCH		DINNER		BEDTIME	
Thursday	BEFORE	AFTER	BEFORE	AFTER	BEFORE	AFTER	BEFORE	AFTER
BLOOD SUGAR								
BLOOD PRESSURE								
Date __/__/__	BREAKFAST		LUNCH		DINNER		BEDTIME	
Friday	BEFORE	AFTER	BEFORE	AFTER	BEFORE	AFTER	BEFORE	AFTER
BLOOD SUGAR								
BLOOD PRESSURE								
Date __/__/__	BREAKFAST		LUNCH		DINNER		BEDTIME	
Saturday	BEFORE	AFTER	BEFORE	AFTER	BEFORE	AFTER	BEFORE	AFTER
BLOOD SUGAR								
BLOOD PRESSURE								
Date __/__/__	BREAKFAST		LUNCH		DINNER		BEDTIME	
Sunday	BEFORE	AFTER	BEFORE	AFTER	BEFORE	AFTER	BEFORE	AFTER
BLOOD SUGAR								
BLOOD PRESSURE								

NOTES: _____
_____
_____

Made in the USA
Columbia, SC
12 July 2022